D1552156

AQUATIC EXERCISE

AQUATIC EXERCISE

BY

RUTH SOVA

SECOND EDITION

DSL, Ltd.
1218 Noridge Trail
Port Washington, WI 53074

Library of Congress Cataloging-in-Publication Data
Sova, Ruth.
  Aquatic exercise / Ruth Sova
  p.   127   cm.
  Includes bibliographical references.
  ISBN 0-86720-754-X
  1. Aquatic exercises.   2. Aquatic exercises – Therapeutic use.
  I.   Title.
  GV838.53.E94S665   1992
  613.7'16—dc20   92-18243
                                                   CIP

First Edition, 1993
  Reprinted 1996
Second Edition, 2000

Production Editor: Ellen Dybdahl, Cheryl Gorton
Copyeditor: Mary Schmit, Kurt Sova
Proofing Editor: Nicole Sova
Design: Cheryl Gorton
Production: DSL, Ltd.
Cover Design: Kurt Sova/Cheri Gorton
Printing and Binding: McNaughton & Gunn, Inc.
Photos: Kurt Sova, Bud Sova, Donna Manzeck
Illustrations: Dave Garacci

Printed in the United States of America

Dedicated to

Bud

In Memory of

my grandparents from England, Germany and Finland
and their pioneering that brought me to where I am

Other books by Ruth Sova:

Ai Chi – Flowing Aquatic Energy
Ai Chi – Balance, Harmony and Healing
Aqua Fit
Aquatics Handbook
AQUATICS – The Complete Reference Guide for Aquatic Fitness Professionals
AQUATICS – Applied Study Guide and Self-Tests for AEA Certification and Recertification
BackHab
Essential Principles of Aquatic Therapy and Rehabilitation
Painless Strategic Planning
Water Fitness After 40

If you're interested in booking Ruth Sova as a speaker please contact:

Aquatic Therapy & Rehab Institute
Route 1 Box 218
Chassell, MI 49916

906-482-4333
Fax 906-482-4388
atri@up.net
www.atri.org

Acknowledgements

Thanks to everyone who's helped me on this journey and especially:

My friend, Ellen Dybdahl, who typed and typed and typed, and shares tea with me.

My husband, Bud Sova, who was no help at all but I'd feel badly leaving him out.

Our son and daughter-in-law, Kurt and Erin Sova, who are fun and always available for photography.

Our daughter and son-in-law, Nicole Sova and Dave Garacci, who have depth beyond their years and pay their own bills.

My sister, Anne Miller, who keeps me in my place while making me strive for excellence.

Mom and my brothers, Paul and John, who support me on this earth, and Dad who's with me always.

My friends, Peggy Bannon and Al Esselmann for their friendship (and their pool) who with Jim and Maria Kiesow and Kevin Ackeret keep me centered and laughing.

My friend, Adolph Kiefer, who has broadened my horizons.

*"Life either polishes you up
or grinds you down."*

The Rev. Dr. R.J. Jalkanen

Preface

...from Ruth Sova

This book will get you started – and keep you going for a long time. Use this book as a guide to get you going. When you have questions check the table of contents and find where the answer might be. When you lack exciting "moves" for your next class throw in a few different moves (or their variations) from the choreography chapter. If you want basic information on a muscle balance, check it out in here.

When you've evolved far enough that this book's not answering questions or giving you any motivation it'll be time to move on to *AQUATICS – The Compete Reference Guide for Aquatic Fitness Professionals.* Until then I hope you smile and have happiness in your heart every time you enter the pool, and a feeling of accomplishment every time you leave it

The most important thing you can do with your pool options is to make choices based on love and acceptance, not fear. I urge my children to do this in all choices in life. So many times we make decisions based on fear (fear of failure, fear of embarrassment, fear that someone will look better or achieve more, that someone else will get the job or the accolades, that someone else will get more money, have a nicer house or car, look better physically, be quicker or smarter, etc.) and these decisions always turn out (whether we're aware of it or not) to be the wrong choices. Instead we must teach ourselves to open our hearts and make decisions based on love and acceptance. Those decisions will always be the right ones. Try it with your work in the pool.

Ruth Sova

P.S. That book for your next step that I mentioned is great. The author? Ruth Sova, of course.

AQUATIC EXERCISE

Table of Contents

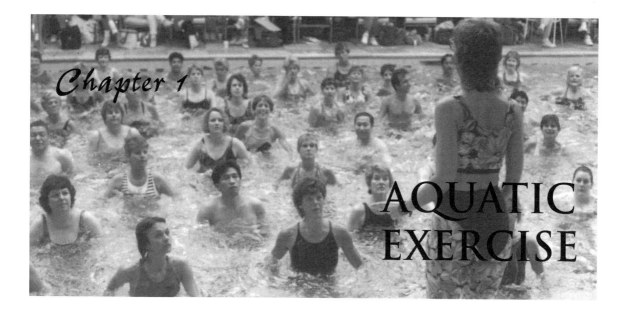

Chapter 1

AQUATIC EXERCISE

Overview

The concept of aquatic exercise is an idea whose time has certainly come. The jogging craze of the late sixties and seventies, the aerobic dance frenzy of the seventies and early eighties, and the pursuit of total fitness through cross training that brought us through the nineties have matured into an intelligent pursuit of health and fitness in the new millennium. Exercise is the fountain of youth, and everyone wants to drink from it.

Like almost everything in life, jogging, aerobic dance, and cross training have proven to be less than perfect. As more people have joined in the bouncing, jumping, jogging, and pumping, reports of minor injuries have become more frequent. The impact experienced during these sports has created countless dropouts. As Baby Boomers move through middle age and become senior citizens, they are demanding a fitness program that will enable them to continue exercising for the rest of their lives, despite the joint problems and reduced flexibility they will eventually experience.

Thus, aquatic exercise has become a major exercise alternative in our fitness-conscious society.

It is a perfect mix of water and workout. Since the movements are performed in chest-deep water, these programs appeal to the swimmer and non-swimmer alike.

The buoyant support of the water effectively cancels approximately 90% of the weight of a person submerged to the neck. This dramatically decreases compression stress on weight-bearing joints, bones, and muscles. Since it is thought that most movements done in the water involve only concentric muscular contractions, muscle soreness is minimal. The possibility of muscle, bone, and joint injuries is almost completely eliminated. Individuals concerned with excess pressure on their ankles, knees, hips, and back can now increase their strength, flexibility, and cardiovascular endurance with safe aerobics: aquatic exercise.

Aquatic exercise is ideal for many people who have painful joints or weak leg muscles and cannot indulge in alternative exercise programs. Special populations—such as those with arthritis or other joint problems, obesity, and back problems, as well as pre- and postnatal women, sedentary individuals, and those recovering from injury or surgery—are prime candidates for aquatic exercise.

With the body submerged in water, blood circulation automatically increases to some extent. Water pressure on the body also helps to promote deeper ventilation (breathing) of the lungs. With a well-planned activity, both circulation and ventilation increase even more.

Flexibility work is increased and performed more easily in water because of the lessened gravitational pull. It is much easier to do leg straddles or side stretches in the water than out. Many individuals can do leg bobbing or jogging in the water who could never do so on land. The resistant properties of water also make it a perfect exercise medium for the well-conditioned individual who is looking to accomplish more in less time. The resistance of the water makes taking a simple walk a challenging workout, testing muscular endurance and strength and cardiorespiratory fitness. Vigorous water exercise can make a major contribution to individual flexibility, muscular strength and endurance, body composition, and cardiorespiratory fitness.

There are many kinds of aquatic exercise programs to choose from. Many are described in this book. Variations can be made by combining or alternating programs to suit an individual's specific needs.

In this book, the term aquatic or water exercise will refer to vertical exercise in the water with the participant submerged to chest or shoulder depth. Most aquatic exercisers stand in chest-deep water or work out vertically in the deep end (diving well) of the pool while using buoyant devices.

Overall Fitness

Overall fitness may be defined as a combination of physical, mental, and emotional well-being. It implies a positive outlook on life with enough strength and stamina to perform the daily tasks of living with energy to spare for leisure pursuits.

Hypokinetic Disease

For reasons we are just beginning to understand, physical fitness is related to overall fitness and total well-being in a variety of ways. Unfortunately, our society continues to be largely sedentary, which conflicts with the inherent purpose of our bodies, namely, that they were designed for movement.

Movement helps to keep us healthy. Without movement, our bodies begin to deteriorate. Sometimes that deterioration is mistakenly chalked up to age instead of disuse. The deterioration that results from inactivity has caused a whole new syndrome of disease in our society, diseases that are hypokinetic. Hypokinetic disease is a condition caused by or aggravated by inactivity. (Hypo means "not enough." Kinetic means "movement.")

Common examples of hypokinetic disease are heart disease, back pain, obesity, ulcers, and blood vessel diseases such as atherosclerosis. Hypokinetic mental disorders include insomnia, lethargy, depression, anxiety, and a sense of unease. Hypokinetic diseases also include metabolic disorders, such as adult-onset diabetes and hypoglycemia; bone and joint disorders, such as osteoporosis and osteoarthritis; and the stress disorders of constipation and mood swings.

The physically fit person, besides having a reduced risk of hypokinetic disease, is more likely than her/his unfit neighbor to feel good, look good, and enjoy life. S/he can work and play more effectively; s/he is more creative; and s/he is less likely to suffer from anxiety, depression, and psychosomatic illness.

Mind and Body

The mind-body connection in overall fitness works in reverse also. That is, the emotionally stable person with a positive attitude will be less likely to suffer from physical diseases. Dr. Thomas McKeown, a prominent English physician, said, "It is now evident that the health of man is determined predominantly, not by medical intervention, but, by his behavior, his food, and the nature of the world in which he finds himself." Many mindful exercise programs have the potential to help treat a number of chronic disease states. Practicing muscular and mental relaxation techniques, visualization, self-responsibility, cognitive concepts, imagery, breathing techniques and positive affirmations will all help in gaining overall fitness.

Mental Attitude

The mental attitude of the regular exerciser is improved not only by a psychological phenomenon but also by a physical one. While the exact effects of powerful hormones called endorphins are not clear yet, they seem to be related to pain, emotions, appetite, the immune system, exercise, and the reproduction system. The feelings of well-being that come with vigorous exercise have been traced to endorphins. They may also have an effect on mental problems. For instance, patients experiencing depression often have low levels of endorphins.

Mental Sharpness

The mind-body connection also correlates with mental sharpness, alertness, and sometimes intelligence. A study published in the Journal of Aging and Physical Activity shows that exercise may reverse many declines in mental functioning that take place as individuals grow older. A study at Purdue University found that after working out three times a week for six months, one group was not only 20% fitter but scored 70% higher in a test of complex decision making.

Overall fitness should be a goal for all people. This book will cover aspects of the physical portion of fitness. It is a guide to achieving physical fitness through water exercise.

Physical Fitness

Major Components of Physical Fitness

There are five major aspects or components of physical fitness:

1. Cardiorespiratory endurance
2. Muscular strength
3. Muscular endurance
4. Flexibility
5. Body composition

When working toward physical fitness, many people include only one or two of these five aspects in their workout plan. All five components are interrelated yet separate enough that a person can be fit in one aspect but not in the others. A truly fit person will include all aspects of physical fitness in his/her workout and will be fit in each one.

Cardiorespiratory Endurance

Cardiorespiratory endurance or fitness involves the ability of the heart and blood to supply the oxygen from the respiratory system to the cells of the body during sustained exercise. To increase this component of physical fitness, aerobic exercise must take place.

In order to be aerobic, the exercise must be continuous, involve the body's large muscles (the quadriceps, hamstrings, and gluteals in the legs and buttocks), last for at least 20 minutes, and work at a perceived exertion level of "somewhat hard" to "hard" or elevate the heartrate into the working zone. To improve cardiorespiratory endurance, an aerobic workout should be repeated at least three times a week. Leaping, kicking, jogging, and walking in the water will increase the

Diagram 1-1 Primary Risk Factors for Coronary Heart Disease

1. Hypertension (high blood pressure)
2. High blood lipids and cholesterol levels
3. Cigarette smoking
4. Obesity (overweight)
5. Family history of heart disease (close blood relative died suddenly before age of 55 or family history of high cholesterol, Marfan's syndrome, or enlarged heart)
6. Atherosclerosis (hardening of the arteries)
7. Diabetes
8. Sedentary lifestyle (lack of physical activity)
9. Stress
10. Age (women, risk greater after menopause; men, risk increases proportionately with age)
11. Sex (men more at risk than women until age of 50-60, then both are equal)

Muscular Strength

Muscular strength is the ability of a muscle to exert great force in a single effort. It is usually attained by lifting weights. To achieve muscular strength, each muscle group works submaximally (about 60% of the maximum ability) for about eight repetitions. After all muscle groups have been worked, the entire workout is repeated once or twice.

Water offers a natural resistance or weight. Paddles, water-tight weights, webbed gloves, and special weight-training equipment can all be used to intensify the force of the workload in the water.

Muscular Endurance

Muscular endurance is the ability of a muscle to repeat a contraction with a moderate workload over a long period of time. Ten to thirty repetitions of any movement build up endurance rather than strength. A workout involving 10 repetitions working each muscle group can be done three times.

Muscular endurance and toning can be achieved sooner with the water's resistance than with endurance workouts on land. Moreover, there is minimal risk of injury due to the cushioning effect of the water.

workload on the cardiorespiratory system so that endurance benefits can be obtained.

Exercise is usually associated with its cardiac benefits. A recent study has shown that lack of exercise may be the single risk factor most clearly associated with future coronary disease. Regular cardiorespiratory exercise has been shown to improve to a variable degree almost all of the commonly accepted risk factors that can be changed: lack of exercise, elevated cholesterol, elevated triglycerides, lowered high-density lipoproteins (HDL), hypertension, smoking, obesity, stress, and diabetes (glucose metabolism). Myocardial efficiency is also markedly improved, as evidenced by decreased resting pulse and decreased heartrate at the same workload during exercise. The effect of exercise on the heart alone makes it a valuable prescription for both physicians and their patients (see Diagrams 1–1 and 1–2).

Diagram 1-2 Secondary Risk Factors for Coronary Heart Disease

1. Asthma or other allergies
2. Arthritis or other joint problems
3. Anxiety
4. Use of medications, alcohol, drugs
5. Current activity
6. Recent surgery
7. Previous difficulty with exercise (chest discomfort, dizziness, extreme breathlessness)
8. Pregnancy status

Flexibility

Flexibility is the ability of limbs to move the joints through a normal range of motion. Flexibility workouts include static stretching of each major muscle group for 30 to 60 seconds. Only muscles should be stretched, not tendons or ligaments.

Due to the lessened effect of gravity in the water, the joints can be moved through a wider range of motion without excess pressure, and long-term flexibility can be achieved.

Body Composition

Body composition is the proportion of fat body mass to lean body mass. It should not be confused with being overweight or underweight, since it does not deal with weight. In fact, eliminating fat body mass and increasing lean body mass may increase the total body weight. A desirable amount of body fat for women is 18% to 20%. The well-conditioned female athlete normally has 16% to 18% body fat. Men should have 10% to 12% body fat. Male athletes usually achieve 7% to 8% body fat.

The average person burns 400 to 600 calories while performing one hour of aerobic exercise. In the water, 77% of the calories burned come from fat stores, thus reducing the fat mass in a body. Muscle tissue (lean body mass) growth is stimulated while moving through the water resistance.

Minor Components of Physical Fitness

Other components of fitness listed by sports physiologists are called minor components or skill-related components. Skill-related fitness is related to performing motor skills, such as playing soccer or walking a tightrope. The skill-related components of physical fitness are:

Speed—the ability to perform a movement in a short period of time

Power—the ability to transfer energy into force at a fast rate (a combination of strength and speed in one explosive action)

Agility—the ability to rapidly and accurately change the position of the entire body

Reaction time—the amount of time elapsed between stimulation and reaction to that stimulation

Coordination—the integration of separate motor activities in the smooth, efficient execution of a task

Balance—the maintenance of equilibrium while stationary or moving (static and dynamic balance).

All of the fitness components, both health-related and skill-related aspects, are trainable; that is, they will show improvement when subjected to appropriate activity.

Principles of Exercise

Six basic principles of exercise must be understood in order to create a sound exercise program:

1. Overload
2. Progressive overload
3. Adaptation
4. Specificity
5. Reversibility
6. Variability

Overload

The overload principle states that if an increase in demands is made on a muscle or system, that body part will respond by adapting to the increase. If adequate rest and good nutrition accompany the overload, there will be an increase in strength or efficiency. Improvement cannot occur unless overload is present. Training occurs by means of the overload principle.

Progressive Overload

Progressive overload is also sometimes called

progressive resistance. It is the principle of gradually increasing overload. If the overload or stress is increased too quickly, injury, pain, or exhaustion may result instead of proper training. "No pain, no gain" is a fallacy. Trying to do too much, too soon paves the way for exhaustion, pain, and possible injury. Only in competitive athletics, where participants are willing to take enormous risks for the possibility of superior performance, does this slogan have any merit, and even then, it is questionable.

All training of exercise programs should follow the principle of progressive overload. Programs should begin at low intensity, short duration, and minimum frequency and gradually increase the overload in each category. Training occurs by means of the overload principle.

Adaptation

Adaptation is also called *training*. It is an improvement in the fitness level that results when the body adapts to overload. Place greater work demands on a muscle (including the heart) than it is used to performing, and it will respond by getting stronger. Stretch a muscle longer than it is accustomed to being stretched, and it will become more flexible. Expose muscles to sustained activity for longer than they are accustomed to, and muscular endurance will increase.

The body will adapt to the stresses or overload placed on it so that an increase in overload can be made. By the same token, if the overload is less than normal for a specific component of fitness, there will be a decrease in that particular component. Keeping the overload at a constant level will maintain the current level of fitness.

Specificity

The principle of specificity states that only the muscle, body part, or system that is being overloaded will adapt and improve. Thus, a stretching program will not improve cardiorespiratory fit-

ness. Just as overload is specific to each component of fitness, it is also specific to each body part. Those muscle groups being overloaded are the only ones that develop. Weight training for the hamstrings will do nothing for the biceps.

In order to see improvements in all the major components of fitness, the program has to be designed specifically to overload each component. In order to have muscle balance in a workout, the workout must be designed to involve all the muscles equally.

Reversibility

Reversibility means that fitness benefits cannot be stored by the body. Several days without a workout means the training level will start to decline. It is generally thought that it takes 12 weeks to improve the fitness level and only 2 weeks to see it decline.

Variability

Variability is a principle that most people ignore. It states that adaptation or fitness improvements are enhanced by varying the intensity, length, or type of workout. Variability adds to the training effect.

The popular fitness concept of cross training uses variability as its foundation. Athletes who have hit fitness plateaus have been able to move to higher levels of fitness through cross training. Rather than do the same fitness activity for every workout, athletes do different types of workouts on different days. Runners can use deep-water running, biking, and water strength training to increase their fitness levels. Swimmers can use cross-country skiing, water walking, and weight lifting. Any change in the type, intensity, or length of the workout will enhance fitness improvements.

Reasons for cross training include:
- an optimal development of all components of physical fitness

- an enhanced motivation toward exercise adherence
- injury prevention due to avoidance of overtraining and development of balance with opposing muscle groups
- effectiveness in weight-loss programs
- an overall increase in general physical fitness

All training or adaptation works on the principle of stressing the body and letting it recover in a stronger form. Too often, exercisers make the mistake of repeating the same workout, day after day. That can stress the same muscles and joints until an injury occurs.

In designing an exercise program to provide maximum physical and mental health benefits, activities to promote all the major components of fitness should be included. Cardiovascular work should be integral to the program, since cardiovascular fitness is most important for total well-being. Strength and flexibility work enable people to perform their daily tasks with ease, as well as help protect them from back pain. Body composition can be favorably altered by endurance and strength training.

Many of the skill-related fitness components can also be included in a basic exercise program. We know that if a person's goal is to improve in a particular sport, training in the specific fitness components and movement coordinations of that sport are necessary for optimum improvement. Nevertheless, it is easy to incorporate into a series of exercise routines movements to improve speed, agility, reaction time, balance, and coordination with a resultant improvement in overall fitness.

Taking time at the end of each exercise session for conscious voluntary relaxation is important. Slow stretches and guided relaxation add a feeling of mental and physical letting go that has also been shown to have important health benefits.

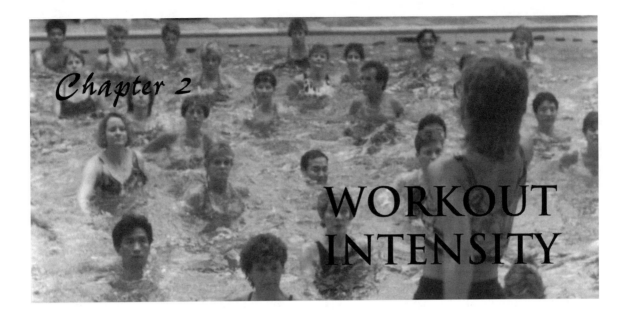

Chapter 2

WORKOUT INTENSITY

Using Heartrate to Measure Intensity

The relationship between heartrate and workout intensity has always been an enigma for aquatic instructors. Many program guidelines advise instructors to check students' exertion levels during class. However, checking heartrates often seems counterproductive. Many students—especially fit ones—are disappointed to learn that their heartrates usually remain lower than the target range recommended to achieve aerobic improvement. Checking perceived exertion doesn't seem to work either because students often don't feel that they have worked as hard in a water exercise class as they have outside running or in a land-based aerobics class.

What's an instructor to do? Exertion levels need to be checked, but doing so sometimes leads students to think that water workouts are wimpy. To help solve this dilemma, instructors must have a thorough understanding of heartrates and their significance in teaching aquatics classes.

Terms and Definitions

Several different terms are used to characterize heartrates:

- Resting heartrate (RHR)
- Maximal heartrate
- Working heartrate range
- Minimum working heartrate
- Maximum working heartrate
- Optimum working heartrate
- Target zone
- Recovery heartrate

Resting Heartrate

The resting heartrate (RHR) is the number of times the heart beats per minute when the body is at rest. This heartrate is usually counted over 60 seconds. The RHR should be measured before getting up in the morning or after 20 minutes of sitting quietly. To ensure an accurate RHR, the exercise participant should measure the resting heartrate on three separate occasions and take the average.

The average resting heartrate is about 72 beats per minute. The RHR of a conditioned adult is often 50 to 60 beats per minute. Lower RHRs generally indicate higher levels of conditioning. Athletes often have resting heartrates of 40 beats per minute or lower. Sedentary or unfit individuals will average resting heartrates of 80 beats per minute or higher.

The RHR is not always a reflection of fitness level. Participants with heart disease will experience lower or higher heartrates at rest and during exercise. People who take beta blockers for hypertension or migraines will also experience lower heartrates. In these conditions, the lowered RHR does not indicate a high fitness level. Caffeine, nicotine, dehydration, tiredness, illness, hot weather, and overtraining can all elevate the resting heartrate. A fit individual whose resting heartrate is higher than usual first thing in the morning should most likely slack off on exercise and allow recovery.

Maximal Heartrate

The maximal heartrate is the greatest number of times per minute the heart is capable of beating. It is the highest heartrate a person can attain during heavy exercise. An accurate measure of the maximal heartrate can be determined by a graded exercise test called a *stress electrocardiogram*. Exercise leaders who do not have access to or the training necessary to do a stress electrocardiogram often calculate maximal heartrate by subtracting the participants age from 220. This number is the general estimation for the maximal heartrate.

Working at or near the maximal heartrate puts great stress on the body; it results in extreme fatigue and does not promote aerobic fitness. The maximal heartrate is often confused with the maximum working heartrate (see following discussion). Students should not work above the maximum working heartrate. Students should not work near the maximal heartrate.

Working Heartrate Range

The working heartrate range is the zone within which an individual needs to work for aerobic training to take place. It is the area between and including the minimum working heartrate and the maximum working heartrate. When the exercising heartrate remains in this zone, cardiorespiratory conditioning is likely to occur. The training intensity range often varies from as little as 50% to 85% of maximal oxygen consumption. A linear relationship exists between heartrate, oxygen consumption, and workload or workout intensity in most land-based exercise situations. Because of that, the *target zone* (target heartrate range or training zone) is used to determine when cardiorespiratory conditioning is occurring during exercise.

Several formulas are currently in use to determine the working heartrate range. The most common (discussed later) are the *maximal heartrate formula* and the *Karvonen formula*.

The top of the target zone, which would be the upper limit of suggested exercise intensity, is the highest percentage. The low percentage is used to determine the minimum threshold to improve cardiorespiratory fitness. The instructor should encourage students who are unfit or just beginning exercise to use the low percentage or to work at or above the minimum working heartrate. As conditioning occurs, students can be encouraged to work at a more comfortable intensity in the middle of the zone. Many internal and external factors affect a participant's heartrate. The instructor should be aware that this zone is merely a guideline. Heartrate will vary from person to person and situation to situation.

Minimum Working Heartrate

Minimum working heartrate is at the low end of the working heartrate range. This is the minimum number of times the heart should beat per minute during exercise for cardiorespiratory training to take place. It is sometimes referred to as the *threshold for aerobic training*. Students should know this number so they can work toward it during exercise.

Maximum Working Heartrate

The maximum working heartrate is at the upper end of the working heartrate range. This is the maximum number of times the heart should beat per minute during exercise for cardiorespiratory training to take place. Working at a level higher than this can be dangerous to individuals with known or unsuspected cardiorespiratory disease and does not promote efficient use of fats for fuel. Working at a rate higher than the maximum working heartrate is considered an anaerobic workout. The maximum working heartrate is often called the *anaerobic threshold*.

Optimum Working Heartrate

Optimum working heartrate is the ideal number of beats per minute for cardiorespiratory training to take place. There are different optimum working heartrates for different fitness goals. The optimum working heartrate always falls between the minimum working heartrate and the maximum working heartrate.

Target Zone

Target zone is another term for the working heartrate range, which is usually 60% to 90% of the maximal heartrate. During a workout, the heartrate should be in the target zone.

Recovery Heartrate

The recovery heartrate is the number of times the heart beats per minute when monitored 5 to 10 minutes after vigorous exercise. It reflects how quickly the cardiorespiratory system is able to return to its preexercise condition. A more fit person will recover faster than a less fit person. The recovery heartrate is often used as an indicator of cardiorespiratory fitness.

Participants who have not recovered to a normal range after five minutes have probably exercised too vigorously and are not conditioned enough to maintain that level for future exercise. They should be cautioned to exercise at a lower intensity during future exercise sessions.

Using Heartrates

It is important to understand heartrate terminology and formulas. Review the previous sections thoroughly to reinforce understanding these concepts.

Scientists have found that the exercising heartrate often correlates closely to oxygen consumption. Based on this correlation, a formula was developed for land-based exercise by a scientist named Karvonen that calculates the heartrate an individual must achieve in order to get desired benefits. The formula is adjusted for age and conditioning level. Aquatic exercisers have begun to adapt it for their fitness programs, as well.

Heartrates can be monitored easily by periodically taking the pulse during an exercise session and then adjusting the exercise intensity to bring the heartrate to the recommended level.

In order to use the formula, exercisers must be taught to monitor their heartrates. Begin by having them place the index and middle fingers on the throat along the carotid artery, pressing lightly. Some exercisers prefer to place the fingers on the wrist at the radial pulse. At either site, the exerciser counts the pulsations while the instructor keeps track of time. While counting, the exerciser should be sure to continue to exercise by walking or jogging in place so that the heartrate doesn't slow down. The thumb should never be used to count pulsation, since it has a pulse of its own.

Formula for Determining Heartrate

The Karvonen formula is a scientific formula commonly accepted as the safest way to calculate the appropriate exertion level for land-based aerobic exercise. It is a relatively accurate and very popular method of determining target heartrate. The Karvonen formula has an error rate of plus or minus 10 beats per minute when used on average individuals in land-based exercise. It is recommended by the American College of Sports Medicine (ACSM).

Since actually measuring the maximal heartrate requires special equipment and trained personnel, the Karvonen formula uses an age-predicted heartrate formula to arrive at the maximal heartrate. The formula is:

220 – age = Maximal heartrate

The age-predicted maximal heartrate formula estimates that 220 is the approximate maximal heartrate of a baby and that each year, this rate decreases by one beat. For example, a 20-year-old

person would have an estimated maximal heartrate of 200 beats per minute (220 – 20 = 200). A 40-year-old would have an estimated maximal heartrate of 180 (220 – 40 = 180). Although this is a commonly used formula, maximal heartrates often vary by plus or minus 10 beats per minute at any given age.

The Karvonen formula then goes on to calculate the *heartrate reserve,* which is the difference between the resting heartrate and the maximal heartrate. This portion of the formula is:

Maximal heartrate
– Resting heartrate
Heartrate reserve

For example, a 40-year-old with a resting heartrate of 60 beats per minute would have a heartrate reserve of 120 (220 – 40 = 180; 180 – 60 = 120).

Once the heartrate reserve has been calculated for each participant, the Karvonen formula becomes simpler. The *target heartrate* equals the heartrate reserve times the percentage of intensity plus the resting heartrate. The training intensity range used in the Karvonen formula is 50% to 85% of maximal heartrate reserve.

For example, a 40-year-old whose resting heartrate is 60 beats per minute is just beginning to exercise regularly and needs to know his or her minimum working heartrate. The heartrate reserve is multiplied by the intensity level, which in this case is 50%, to determine the minimum working heartrate plus the resting heartrate of 60 beats per minute (120 x .50 + 60 = 120). The minimum working heartrate for this exerciser is 120 beats per minute. The maximum working heartrate is determined in the same fashion, but 85% is used for intensity level (120 x .85 + 60 = 162). The maximum working heartrate for this exerciser is 162 beats per minute. The target zone for the exerciser is from 120 to 162 beats per minute.

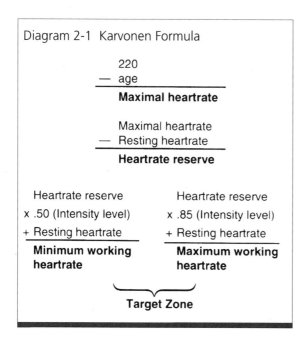

Diagram 2-1 Karvonen Formula

Heartrate, Oxygen, and Caloric Consumption

Some students in aquatics classes feel they don't get as good a workout in the water as they do on land. They are definitely wrong. They need education on heartrate, oxygen consumption, and caloric consumption.

Many students judge the intensity of a workout and thus the value of a class by the heartrate they achieve. If their heartrate is up, they're getting a good workout; if it isn't, they're not. Their mistake is that they assume that heartrate is always an indication of workout intensity. This is not necessarily true. Target heartrates are valid indicators of intensity only if they correlate with oxygen consumption. Because we are aerobic beings, physiologists measure workout intensity or energy expenditure by measuring how much oxygen is utilized by the body during a given activity compared with how much oxygen is used at rest.

A given pace of exercise requires a specific amount of oxygen utilization. One quart of oxygen utilization equals 5 calories. If a participant wanted to work at a 10-calorie-per-minute pace, s/he would need 2 quarts of oxygen per minute. The average outdoor walker uses 5 calories per minute, which would be 1 quart of oxygen per minute. The average outdoor jogger uses 10 calories per minute or 2 quarts per minute.

This information can make it simple for students to understand that caloric consumption is tied to oxygen consumption or utilization, not to heartrate. Heartrate is not always indicative of the amount of calories being burned. If caloric consumption is the exerciser's goal, s/he should increase his or her oxygen consumption, not necessarily his or her heartrate.

Unfortunately, oxygen consumption is measured with expensive, technical, cumbersome equipment that is attached to the exerciser with a breathing apparatus. It's impossible for exercisers outside a laboratory to check oxygen consumption.

That brings us back to heartrate. Heartrate is checked instead of oxygen consumption simply because everyone can do it easily. Formulas have been devised to correlate heartrate almost exactly to oxygen consumption if all conditions are ideal. Many land-based exercises, like running, biking, and aerobics, have almost ideal conditions and can use heartrate as their guide for workout intensity level.

Aquatic Heartrate

Students who participate in both land- and water-based exercise often find their heartrates lower from water exercise than land exercise, yet they receive the same benefits. There are no conclusive studies as to why this happens. There are, however, several commonly accepted theories.

Theories for Variations

1. *Heat*—When exercising, the body creates excess heat. One of the functions of the circulatory system is to dissipate heat from the body. Because water dissipates heat more effectively than air, the heart may not beat as fast as it does on land to cool the body. Cooler water temperature will lower the heart rate response.
2. *Gravity*—Water lessens the effect of gravity on the body, and improves venous return which lowers the heart rate.
3. *Compression*—Water is a subtle compression on the veins and arteries which facilitates bloodflow back to the heart while exercising, reducing stress on the heart and resulting in a lower working heartrate.
4. *Partial pressure*—Oxygen is absorbed more easily into the blood during aquatic exercise which may reduce the workload of the heart.
5. *Dive reflex*—When the body is submerged, this reflex lowers heartrate and blood pressure.

To compensate for the observed reduction in

heartrate during water-based exercise, a variety of techniques are being used. A study done at the Human Performance Lab at Adelphi University found that even though water-based heartrates were reported to be 13% lower than the land-based minimum and maximum counts, the cardiorespiratory benefits were the same as those produced by land-based exercise. The Institute for Aerobics Research in Dallas, Texas, deducts 17 beats per minute from their projected heartrates for water exercise. The 17-beat deduction was also verified in horizontal water exercise and documented by McArdle, Katch, and Katch in *Exercise, Physiology, Energy, Nutrition, and Human Performance*. A 14% decrease in water heart rates was shown in a 1996 study and a 1990 study showed a 10 to 12-beat reduction in the heart rate of sedentary subjects.

While observation has shown that heartrates are generally lower in aquatic exercise, clearly more studies are needed. Until then, heartrate information must be accepted as a basic guide rather than a hard-and-fast rule for measuring exercise intensity.

Applying Variations to the Karvonen Formula

Applying this information to the Karvonen formula, consider once again a prospective exerciser who is 40-years-old and has reported a resting heartrate of 60 beats per minute (see earlier examples). The final target zone of working heartrates for water exercise would be from 103 to 145 beats per minute. This range is determined by subtracting 17 from the original land-based figures for minimum and maximum working heartrates. Namely, the minimum working heartrate for land-based exercise was 120 beats per minute and the maximum, 162 beats per minute. The target zone for water-based exercise is 103 to 145 beats per minute.

Student Variations

Common sense must prevail when monitoring heartrate. There is a percentage of students for whom the technique and formula will not be accurate. This may be due to medications or specific disease conditions, both chronic and acute. Instructors should familiarize these students with other subjective measures of exercise intensity, such as the perceived exertion scale, the "talk test," and respiration rate so that they can be used in the place of heartrate monitoring.

Instructors should observe each student for signs of overexertion, such as shortness of breath, excessively red or splotchy skin color, excessive sweating, or excessive fatigue. If these symptoms are observed, exercise should be stopped by gradually cooling down, and the student should be

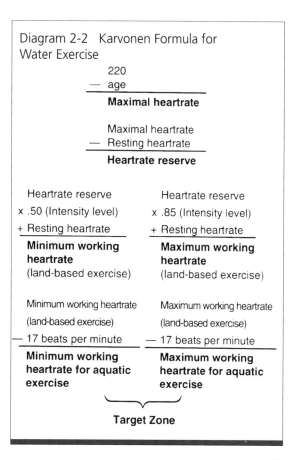

referred to a doctor.

Recovery heartrates following exercise are considered safe when recorded at 110 beats per minute or lower. If a student's heartrate is still above 110, encourage him or her to continue exercising at a low level, and check the heartrate again after a few minutes. The student should not leave the pool or be left unsupervised until the heartrate is below 110 beats per minute.

If a student consistently takes a long time to recover from aerobics, advise him or her to use a slightly slower, less strenuous pace throughout the workout. Continue to check the recovery heartrate. If the pattern continues, advise the student to notify his or her doctor.

Alternate Intensity Evaluation Methods

Clearly many factors—from exercising in shallow water or high humidity to wearing restrictive clothing to taking medications—will increase the heartrate. Unfortunately, students often try to use these factors when trying to increase the intensity of a workout. But so often in aquatic exercise, the true intensity of the workout (oxygen consumption) and heartrate do not correlate at all. Because of this, instructors should be familiar with alternative methods of evaluating exercise intensity, which include subjective measurements such as perceived exertion, respiration rate, and the "talk test."

Rate of Perceived Exertion

While heartrate isn't always a good indicator of intensity, exercisers are. Exercise physiologists working with a scientist named Gunnar Borg discovered that exercisers are able to sense their own intensity levels. Participants are asked to label their activities as "Very, very light;" "Very light;" "Fairly light;" "Somewhat hard;" "Hard;" "Very hard;" or "Very, very hard." Participants are able to closely approximate their heartrate readings by how hard they perceive themselves to be working.

Based on Borg's rate of perceived exertion (RPE) chart included (see Diagram 2–3), most exercisers should be working in the "Somewhat hard" to "Hard" range. "Very, very light" describes feelings of exertion at total rest, and "Very, very hard" describes feelings just before collapsing of exhaustion. The numbers in the left-hand column correspond to a 6-second land-based exercise heartrate.

Pollock, Wilmore, and Fox found that ratings of 12 to 13 are equal to about 60% of maximal heartrate reserve, while 16 is equal to about 90% of maximal heartrate reserve. Participants working in the

Diagram 2-3 Borg's Rate of Perceived Exertion (RPE) Chart	
6	
7	Very, very light
8	
9	Very light
10	
11	Fairly light
12	
13	Somewhat hard
14	
15	Hard
16	
17	Very hard
18	
19	Very, very hard
20	

Source: Borg, G. A. V. (1982). Psychophysical Bases of Physical Exertion. *Medicine and Science in Sport and Exercise, 14,* 344–387. Used with permission.

Diagram 2-4 American College of Sports Medicine (ACSM) Rate of Perceived Exertion (RPE) Chart

0	Nothing
0.5	Very, very light (just noticeable)
1.0	Very light
2	Light (weak)
3	Moderate
4	Somewhat hard
5	Heavy (strong)
6	
7	Very heavy
8	
9	
10	Very, very heavy (almost max)

tensity in cardiovascular activity. In fact, some exercise professionals find it to be the most useful indicator of workout intensity. Some aquatic exercise instructors combine heartrate response and RPE methods. They have participants get used to taking a pulse during exercise and relating to how they feel during that workout. After a few weeks of pulse checks, participants are able to perceive their own levels of intensity without checking pulses.

Estimated Time Limit

Researchers at the Laboratoire de Physiolgie du Travail et du Sport in La Pitie Salpetriere, France, have tried to further quantify Borg's Rating of Perceived Exertion (RPE). They propose a 20-point logarithmic scale of perceived exertion that measures "Estimated Time Limit" (ETL), or how long the exerciser thinks he can continue to exercise at that intensity before exhaustion. Aerobic exercisers shooting for 40 percent of their VO_2 max are looking at an ETL of 5 (exhaustion in four hours) to 12 (exhaustion in 23 minutes).

ETL corresponds well with heart rate, maximal aerobic power, VO_2 max and Borg's RPE, at least

"Somewhat hard" to "Hard" range during the aerobic phase of the class will be working in the 60% to 90% range of maximal heartrate reserve.

Borg found that the RPE scale correlated very highly with heartrate, ventilation, oxygen consumption, and blood lactate concentration. Since it has already been shown that heartrate is not a very reliable measure of exertion in aquatic exercise, it seems that the RPE method may work well not only for aquatic exercisers but for all of the special populations using medications.

The ACSM revised the RPE scale in 1986 to make it simpler for participants to use (see Diagram 2–4). This scale goes from 0, which is "Nothing," to 10, which is "Very, very heavy." It provides more verbal descriptions for participants to use in rating their exertion levels.

Participants in water exercise sometimes perceive their exertion to be somewhat lower because of the cooling effect and the enjoyment of the water. This is not the case, however. The RPE method can be a reliable guide to measuring in-

Diagram 2-5 Estimated Time Limit

ETL	TIME UNTIL EXHAUSTION
20	Less than 2 minutes
19	2 minutes
17	4 minutes
15	8 minutes
13	15 minutes
11	30 minutes
9	1 hour
7	2 hours
5	4 hours
3	8 hours
1	More than 16 hours

International Journal of Sports Medicine,
January 1999:20: 40-42

in low and moderate exercise intensity. ETL is less reliable at exercise intensity levels above the ventilatory anaerobic threshold, which occurred at ETL=10 (exhaustion in 45 minutes), and RPE=15 ("hard").

Respiration Rate

In order for an exerciser to get extra oxygen, s/he must take more breaths per minute. If the respiration rate (or breaths per minute) during activity doesn't increase, the exercise isn't intense enough. Measuring respiration rate is technique to determine just the lower limit (minimum working heartrate) of intensity.

Therapeutic respiration rate can be characterized by using the dyspnea scale, as follows:

1. Mild—noticeable to exerciser but not to observer
2. Some difficulty—noticeable to observer
3. Moderate difficulty—exerciser can still continue
4. Severe difficulty—exerciser cannot continue

Dyspnea is defined as shortness of breath or labored breathing. Using respiration rate to determine exercise intensity is normally done in conjunction with another method, such as heartrate or RPE, for monitoring intensity.

"Talk Test"

The so-called "talk test" is very simple: If participants can't talk when they're exercising, it means they're working too hard. If they are working out so strenuously that they can't visit with the person next to them, it means the exercise is no longer aerobic. Participants should be able to breathe comfortably and deeply during the entire workout. If they are short of breath, panting, or gasping and are unable to talk, their workout is too intense. Rather than burning fat and carbohydrate

calories, they are burning protein. The "talk test" monitors only the top end of the target zone (maximum working heartrate).

Increasing Intensity

Participants often think they're getting a great workout in warm, shallow water, with their arms overhead and the sun shining. As most instructors know, heartrates are probably only elevated because of heart stress, not increased oxygen or caloric consumption.

If exercisers are too concerned with achieving a specific heartrate, they may injure themselves in an effort to burn many calories. And ironically, they may actually not burn as many calories as they might with a more sensible program and a lower heartrate or perceived exertion rate. In these instances, the heartrate may not be in an average target range, but the oxygen consumption may be high enough to burn calories at a level as though the heartrate were in the target range. This is what was found with the research discussed earlier.

If participants feel they're not working hard enough, they can increase their intensity level by experimenting with a few of the concepts listed below. They'll be able to tell what makes them "huff and puff," namely, increasing oxygen consumption. If they're not breathing harder and deeper after the warm-up, they're not working hard enough. (Kicks are used as an example since almost all programs include them during a workout.)

1.   Put a big bounce between every kick. Students should push up off the bottom of the pool as hard as they can to get the body high out of the water.

2.   Delete the bounce completely. Have students use only muscle power to kick the leg as high as they can and then return it from the kick. The rest of the body should stay in good postural

alignment. The top part of the body should barely move. This will increase the demand for oxygen in the leg muscles.

3.   Move through the water during the kicks. Participants can move forward and backward or to the corners and back. Moving the body through the resistance of the water will increase the body's oxygen demands.

4.   Move further through the water than usual. If students usually can move four feet forward in eight kicks, challenge them to move five feet forward in eight kicks. This will force more muscle fibers into action and therefore increase the oxygen consumption.

5.   Lift the kicks higher. Push participants to achieve the largest range of motion possible in the time allotted to do each kick. These should be done without jerking at the joint, moving out of alignment, or leaning forward.

6.   Add some force or muscle power to the arm movements that are being used with the kicks. The more muscles involved, the more oxygen will be required. Students should get their arms working, too.

7.   Do the kicks faster. Increasing the speed while still maintaining a safe, upright body alignment can increase the intensity. Students should not, however, compromise the joint by increasing the speed too much. If there's any joint stress, skip this hint and use only numbers 1 through 6 and 8.

8.   Do the kicks slower. Slower kicks (again, done only with good postural alignment) will allow students to use a fuller range of motion (higher kicks) and concentrate on using muscles on the lifting and lowering portions of the kick.

Students need to personally challenge themselves at each class. The instructor's job is to offer a safe, effective, muscle-balanced workout and to help motivate each student. The student's job is to accept the challenge and do a little more at every class. Without adequate effort on the part of the individual, no exercise program will work.

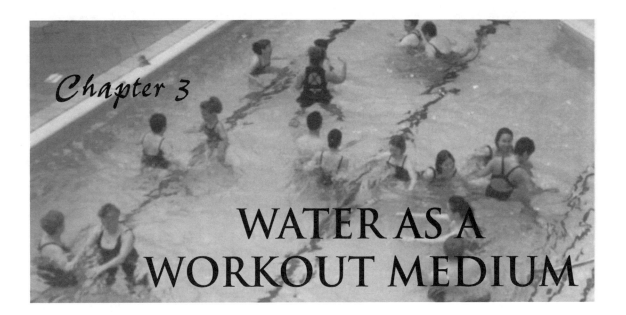

Chapter 3

WATER AS A WORKOUT MEDIUM

General Information

Because of water's unique properties, water-based exercise will provide somewhat different benefits than land-based exercise. To allow for those properties, modifications need to be made before using land-based exercises in the water.

Water Resistance

Water has approximately 12 times the resistance of air. That resistance may slow the exerciser down, but it gives him or her some tremendous benefits.

Movement Speed

When moving in the water, exercisers will need to modify the pace of the movements to allow for the water resistance. The speed of the movements must be adjusted so they can be accomplished without jerking or compromising alignment and using a full range of motion. Movements should always be controlled. If the exercise being done causes the body to move out of alignment in an uncontrolled fashion, it is too fast. The speed at

which one would jog on land is not the speed at which one should jog in the water. Likewise, the speed of kicks done on land should not be used for kicks done in the water. Moving through the water with ballistic, land-based speed movements can cause injuries to the joints and ligaments.

Toning Potential

Water resistance, while slowing an exerciser down, will also provide excellent benefits. While moving through the water, one will not only receive cardiovascular benefits (by pushing the heartrate or perceived exertion level up into the target zone); one will also receive toning benefits not available on land. The water resistance acts with equalized pressure on all body parts that are submerged. Any time a limb is moved through the water, additional toning is created because more muscle fibers are recruited to accommodate the water resistance.

Water as a Workout Medium

Muscle Balance

Muscle balance is another benefit of working in the water. Almost all of the joints in the body have some muscles that flex them and other muscles that extend them. The two muscles that work a joint (flex and extend) are generally thought of as a pair, or muscle pair. The flexors are almost always stronger than the extensors. The extensors generally work with gravity, which does the work for them; thus, extensors are not usually well developed. If exercise programs contribute to the muscle imbalance already developed, injury could result, especially if those joints are weight bearing.

When participants exercise in the water, they are able to get equalized muscle balance that is not available through any other medium. Due to the flotation effect of water, a person working vertically in the water will use the iliopsoas (hip flexor) muscles when lifting (kicking forward) the leg and will get the additional benefit (not received on land) of using the gluteals and hamstrings when lowering the leg back through the water. The same is true with the bicep and tricep muscle pair and most other muscle pairs in the body. While the tricep gets virtually no work during arm extensions in land-based exercises (gravity does the work), water resistance forces the tricep to work when arm extensions are done in the water. Muscle balance is a tremendous benefit of water exercise.

Energy Expenditure

A water workout can give a greater energy expenditure for a workout than a similar land-based exercise would. When walking outside, each step recruits a certain amount of muscle fibers. Each muscle fiber needs a certain amount of oxygen to keep it going. Oxygen consumption correlates with energy and caloric consumption. When the same walking is done in the water rather than on land, more muscle fibers need to be recruited for each step the exerciser takes. That means more

oxygen will be used, and there will be a greater energy and caloric expenditure.

Water-based exercise can achieve a workout intensity similar to that of land-based exercise with less heart stress. One of the functions of the heart is to help the body dissipate heat. If the heart has to work at dissipating heat at the same time it is working to deliver oxygen to the muscles, it can become overloaded and work at a higher rate (beats per minute) than necessary for cardiovascular fitness. If the body is cooled by the water and the heart does not have to work at dissipating heat, it is able to concentrate on simply supplying oxygen to the muscles. Thus, a similar workout intensity is achieved while maintaining a lower heartrate.

Arm Movements

Arm movements in aquatic exercise can be used in much the same way they are used on land: for variety and fun, for balance, for coordination improvement, and to add intensity to the workout. In addition, arm movements can be used for other purposes more particularly suited to aquatic exercise.

Arm movements can be used to help the body move through the water. By pressing the hands from front to back, the exerciser is propelled forward. By starting with the arms to the right and sweeping left, the participant slides to the right. If the hands are pushed straight down, the body will spring upward. Each of these movements can be reversed for the opposite effect.

The benefit of using arms to assist with movement in the water becomes especially apparent when the body presents a large surface area and is therefore resistant to the movement. For example, when the participant is facing straight forward and attempts to jump ahead through the water, the frontal resistance of the body is at its greatest. It is extremely difficult to accomplish this movement without using the arms. As one jogs through the water, more territory can be covered if arms are added to the movement to help pull the body forward.

Changing directions can produce swirls of water, which make movement more difficult. Appropriate arm movements can assist the body in accomplishing direction changes.

In the water, when the body is at a standstill, it takes more effort to put it into motion than it does to maintain a standstill. Upper-body movements can add to the total effort and make it possible to overcome this resistance.

All the while arms are being used in the water for balance, coordination, movement assists, or fun, they are also developing muscular endurance and strength in the upper body. The pushing, pulling, sweeping, flicking, and lifting all work the muscles in the upper and lower arms, the shoulders, the chest, the abdominals, and the upper and lower back. If arms are kept submerged while executing the movements, the potential for gains is even greater, as the water resistance acts like weights or bands to increase the difficulty of the exercise. While some movements done out of the water are advantageous for the students and assure that the joint is moved through the full range of motion, the benefits of using the arms in the water to increase the workload should not be overlooked.

The position of the hands and upper body can increase or decrease the intensity of various exercises. Because swimming programs train people to move efficiently in the water, it is sometimes difficult for them to learn to purposely increase the water resistance to make a workout more difficult.

Presenting a small surface area against the water makes arm movements easier to perform. For example, turning the hands so that they slice through the water requires less effort from the upper body than if the hands are flattened to the direction of the movement. By choosing the appropriate hand position for each movement, aquatic exercisers can do one movement but develop different degrees of conditioning, depending on the workload they place on the muscle.

In addition to affecting the particular muscles in use, arm movements can affect the cardiorespiratory demands on the body during exercise. Greater demand is placed on the heart and lungs as they work harder to meet the muscles' needs for oxygen, nutrients, and waste removal. This is accomplished simply by adding arm movements rather than letting arms hang in the water. Cardiorespiratory conditioning can be boosted even further by cupping or flattening the hands as the arms move through the water.

Water Buoyancy and Cushioning

The cushioning effect is another benefit of exercise in the water. Because of the 90% apparent weight loss in shoulder-depth water, participants are able to exercise with less biomechanical stress during each footstrike or impact. This allows them to exercise longer and more frequently and to gain more benefits without the likelihood of injury.

Three concepts regarding buoyancy will affect instructors in aquatic exercise programming: buoyancy assisted, buoyancy resisted, and buoyancy supported.

1. *Buoyancy assisted* describes a movement that is assisted by buoyancy. This will occur when the move is in the same direction as the force of buoyancy. When a student lifts his or her arm up to the water surface, the force of buoyancy assists that movement. Likewise, when a student lifts his or her leg toward the surface of the water, that movement is buoyancy assisted.

2. *Buoyancy supported* describes a movement that is perpendicular to the force of buoyancy. In this instance, the water simply supports the body or the extremity. A participant standing in the water is experiencing buoyancy support.

3. *Buoyancy resisted* describes a movement

that opposes the force of buoyancy. Returning limbs from flexion to extension or anatomical position is a buoyancy-resisted movement. When a student lifts his or her leg toward the water surface, the movement is being assisted by the force of buoyancy because it is moving in the same direction as that force. While the limb is near the surface of the water, it is being supported by the force of buoyancy, as is the rest of the body in a vertical position. When the leg is returned to the beginning position, the muscles must work harder because it is a buoyancy-resisted movement. Returning the limb to anatomical position opposes the force of buoyancy.

In short, anything moving up toward the surface of the water will be buoyancy assisted. Anything moving down through the water will be buoyancy resisted.

Hydrostatic Pressure

Hydrostatic pressure is the pressure exerted by any fluid on any body at rest. Since there is no resting position in water, some scholars believe that the synergistic and fixator muscles must constantly act to stabilize the body. This pressure is equal on all surfaces of the body; however, it increases with the depth of the water. At the surface, the hydrostatic pressure is 14.7 pounds per square inch. For every added foot of depth, the hydrostatic pressure increases by .433 pounds per square inch. This pressure causes venous blood to return to the heart easily rather than to pool in the lower body, causing lower heartrates in aquatic exercise than land-based exercise without losing aerobic benefits.

Summary

Understanding the water principles that affect participants as they work in the water is important to aquatic exercise instructors. With such knowledge, instructors will be able to increase or decrease the workout intensity for each partici-

pant in a safe, logical manner.

However, instructors must remember that none of these water principles acts individually. A combination of forces will always be at work, affecting the participant's movement in the water. Understanding each principle individually will give the instructor the knowledge base to understand how they interact and provide students with the best exercise program.

Pool Conditions

Knowledge about the area where water exercise classes meet will help the instructor ensure a safe program for participants. Different programs will be ideally suited to different pool environments. Being aware of the factors that are not ideal will allow the instructor to modify conditions and compensate for inadequacies.

Pool Bottom

While aquatic exercise is virtually stress and injury free, the type of pool bottom can affect the likelihood of injury. Slippery pool bottoms can easily cause injuries. Participants whose feet slide out from under them while exercising can injure muscles and ligaments in their legs and backs. Painted pool bottoms or pools done completely in tile or fiberglass or with tile lane markers will be especially slippery. Exercisers encountering a slippery pool bottom should wear some type of footwear that provides traction. The Aquatic Consulting Services suggest .6 as a minimum friction coefficient for pool bottoms.

The pool bottom should have a smooth but nonslippery surface. It should be marked plainly and conspicuously to indicate depth, with specific markings at break points. The proper grate on the drain cover should be screwed in.

Rough pool bottoms can often cause undue wear and tear on the skin of the feet. Exercisers should use some type of protective footwear in the pool if they are losing more than a superficial layer of skin from the bottoms of their feet. Exercisers whose feet have open sores from a rough pool bottom should not be allowed back into the pool until the feet have healed.

Sloped pool bottoms are often dangerous because they create an imbalance in the exercising body, which in turn creates poor postural alignment. Having one foot slightly higher than the other or either the toes or heels higher can eventually lead to an overuse injury. Pools with extreme slopes should not be used or should be used only for deep-water exercise. If an exerciser has to work in a pool with a mild slope, he should move to new areas of the pool and turn in different directions so that the footstrike isn't always off balance in exactly the same way. Most pools of depths of 5 feet or less are sloped at ratios of 1:8 (a one-foot slope for every eight feet of pool bottom) or 1:12, depending on state codes. Depths of over five feet usually have a slope ratio of 1:3.

Water Temperature

The average indoor pool temperature ranges from the high 70s to the low 90s (degrees Fahrenheit). Outdoor pool temperatures can range from the 40s to over 100 degrees.

The temperature of the water is of utmost importance. For high-intensity workouts with healthy, fit individuals who need to dissipate heat, ideal pool temperatures should be 80 to 84 degrees Fahrenheit. In water below 80 degrees, participants must increase the time spent in the warm-up phase before moving on to full-range-of-motion, high-level aerobic activity.

Even when it is within this ideal temperature range, pool water is cooler than body temperature, and it will cause certain physiological reactions to occur: the blood vessels near the surface of the skin will become much smaller; blood will circulate more in the deep vessels of the body in

an attempt to conserve body heat; the muscles will automatically contract; and the participant may begin to shiver. Because of these natural reactions, it is essential that exercisers begin moving immediately upon entering the water. The thermal warm-up should have participants bouncing, jogging, and jazzkicking from the moment of immersion. Continuous motion must be maintained as the workout progresses and the exerciser begins to burn nutrients; this compensates for the heat that is lost to the cool water enveloping the body.

A body in water cools down approximately four times faster than a body in air. Even during a brief pause, the body's temperature can drop enough to cause muscle tightening. During leg, gluteal, and hip-flexor stretches, the arms should continue to move in order to generate body heat. While the exerciser stretches the upper body, the feet should keep marching or jogging. Because of these physiological responses to cool water, a few instructors prefer to do the poststretch on the pool deck.

On occasion the pool temperature will be too cold to enable participants to warm-up adequately and participate safely in an aquatic exercise program. Although the exact water temperatures will vary with different types of students, water temperature in the low 70s and under will likely provide an unsafe exercise environment.

While cool temperatures present one set of difficulties, pools with temperatures over 85 degrees present another potential risk, that of overheating. Warm water interferes with the body's ability to radiate excess heat to a cooler environment; overheating may result. Caution is needed. Many therapeutic pools are heated to over 90 degrees. These pools should not be used for aerobic activities.

Water temperature minimums and maximums are also sometimes set by state, county, or city bathing codes. The temperature should be conducive to the types of activities being offered in the pool.

Water Depth

When choosing appropriate water depth, different considerations should be made regarding the body type of the exerciser and the goal of the program: whether upper-body toning is a priority (if the arms are submerged, more upper-body toning will occur), how much control of movements is possible, whether a good sense of balance can be achieved, and how much safety from impact can be ensured.

The ideal water depth for most aquatic exercisers is between midriff and armpit. This water depth allows participants to use their arms in the water to allow for additional body toning. They will also be able to experience enough body weight to have control of their movements, keep a good sense of balance, and maintain reasonable footing during the exercises. Midriff to armpit water depth also allows the exerciser to experience enough body weight to make the workout a challenge and achieve the intensity needed to produce cardiovascular benefits. At that depth, however, participants will be able to experience enough buoyancy to protect their joints, ligaments, and tendons from the stress of high impact.

Sun Exposure

Instructors and students who work in outdoor pools are placed at unusually high risk for skin cancer if they are regularly exposed to the sun's direct or indirect rays. The American Cancer Society says that the risk is compounded by the fact that exposure is both to sunlight and potent UV reflections off the water surface. Skin cancer is almost entirely preventable if participants and instructors take necessary precautions. Wearing a wide-brimmed hat, using sunscreen or sunblock, and working out before 11 a.m. or after 2 p.m. will help protect the skin from the sun.

Eye safety is also an important consideration for instructors working outdoors. Instructors should wear protective eyewear to prevent corneal sunburn.

Lighting

Lighting should be adequate in the pool area, as well as in the pool and overhead. The glare from natural or artificial lighting should not interfere with visibility. All lights should be functional and protected. Past laws required lighting of 3-1/2 to 4 watts per square foot. New recommendations are given in terms of illumination. Lighting requirements on the deck are 100 lumens (foot candles) per square foot at the water surface. Water surface lighting requirements for outdoor pools are 60 lumens per square foot.

Current Operating License

The current operating license or permit for public pools should be posted in public view. Pool rules and information should also be posted in a conspicuous place. A safety orientation should be provided for new members.

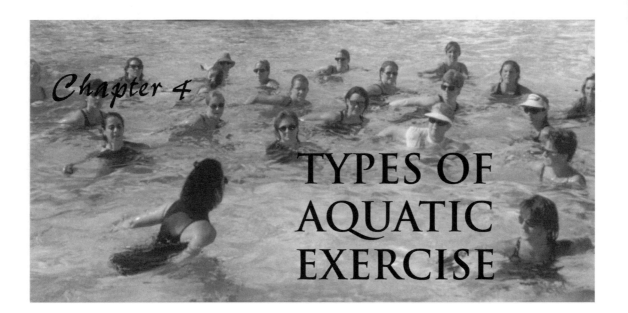

Chapter 4

TYPES OF AQUATIC EXERCISE

The format of aquatic exercise programs will vary, depending on the goals or purposes they have. Almost any program or program variation will follow the aerobic or nonaerobic class format. Programs focusing on cardiorespiratory conditioning (water aerobics, water walking, deep-water programs, circuit training, etc.) follow the *aerobic* class format. Programs that focus on muscular endurance, strength, or flexibility follow the *nonaerobic* class format.

Format for Cardiorespiratory-Conditioning Classes

Warm-Up

Water cardiorespiratory (aerobic) classes usually begin with a warm-up lasting 5 to 10 minutes. Three types of warm-ups needed for program safety: the musculoskeletal warm-up (called the thermal warm-up), the prestretch, and the cardiorespiratory warm-up.

Thermal Warm-Up

The warm-up portion begins with a thermal warm-up. The thermal warm-up is aimed at the skeletal muscles (those on the surface of the body that make you move) and the bones that support them. It involves gentle movements, done with control, using a small range of motion that is gradually increased. This part of the warm-up is designed to bring increased bloodflow to the muscles and soft tissues surrounding the joints, to increase the internal body temperature, and to release synovial fluid.

During the thermal warm-up, the internal body temperature should increase one to two degrees. The raised muscle temperature is ideal for the chemical reactions that occur when exercising vigorously. The raised temperature also makes muscle fibers more pliable, which reduces the likelihood of injury when kicking, jogging, pushing, and pulling during a vigorous workout.

Joints benefit from the thermal warm-up, as well. When movement occurs, synovial fluid is released which helps the joint glide rather than grind.

The thermal warm-up should last approximately three to five minutes. Major muscle groups should be used in the same manner in which they will be used during the aerobic portion of the workout. All major muscle groups and joints should be used in isolation exercises and low- to moderate-intensity exercises. Beginning slowly, with short levers and a reduced range of motion, will stimulate the release of synovial fluid to lubricate the joints and allow the body to gradually warm up. The later portion of the thermal warm-up can incorporate movements with a fuller range of motion, long levers, and more powerful contractions of each muscle group.

Prestretch

A prestretch segment, the next part of the warm-up, is designed to prevent injury during the high-intensity workout to come. Stretching muscles that are tight from everyday living is important. While any of the major muscle groups can be stretched at this point, the gastrocnemius and soleus (calf), iliopsoas (hip flexors), hamstrings (back of the thigh), low-back, and pectoral (chest) muscles should all be stretched during this portion of the workout. Stretches are usually held for 5 to 10 seconds during the prestretch.

Cardiorespiratory Warm-Up

The cardiorespiratory warm-up is the last portion of the warm-up and includes exercises with an increased range of motion and more moderate intensity. The purpose of the cardiorespiratory warm-up is to gradually overload the heart, lungs, and vascular system. It is safest and most efficient to allow all parts to gradually adjust to the increased demands. This is true for all the systems in the body.

This part of the warm-up further increases the oxygen demands on the heart and elevates the core temperature of the body. (Muscle temperature may increase as much as four degrees Fahrenheit during the entire warm-up portion.) The cardiorespiratory warm-up usually lasts three to five minutes.

In order to keep body temperature up during the prestretch segment, some instructors intersperse moves using (and warming) a muscle group and stretching for that muscle group.

Some aquatic exercisers feel that a warm-up is unnecessary or too time consuming for their workouts. Research has shown that beginning a workout with high-intensity, vigorous exercise abnormally increases arterial blood pressure, which in turn causes heart stress. Other research has shown that warming up before a workout significantly reduces abnormal electrocardiograph readings during the vigorous phase as compared to workouts where the participant did not warm up first. These findings prove that a warm-up is important to the safety of participants.

In conclusion, an effective warm-up will produce many benefits; namely, it will:

- increase muscle fluidity, which improves contraction efficiency
- increase the force and rate of muscle contraction
- improve muscle elasticity and the sensitivity of the stretch reflex
- increase the flexibility of tendons, which reduces the risk of injury
- improve metabolic reactions in the muscle that promote more efficient use of carbohydrates and fats
- increase maximal oxygen intake rate and worktime to exhaustion

The Cardiorespiratory Workout

The aerobic portion of the workout is considered the "calorie-burning" portion. The goal of this portion is to improve the cardiorespiratory system. The American College of Sports Medicine (ACSM) has made recommendations for the quantity and quality of training for developing and maintaining cardiorespiratory fitness, body composition and muscular strength, and endurance in the healthy adult. These guidelines address the following aspects of an aerobic exercise (cardiorespiratory) workout:

1. the *mode* —the type of exercise necessary
2. the *duration* —the length of each workout
3. the *intensity* —how challenging the workout is for the cardiorespiratory system
4. the *frequency* —how many times a week the workout should be repeated

If the workout does not follow the guidelines for each of these four aspects, it is not considered to be a cardiorespiratory or aerobic workout.

Mode

The ACSM guidelines state that in order to create the overload necessary to achieve cardiorespiratory fitness, the mode must be a large-muscle activity that is maintained continuously and is rhythmical in nature. This means that the large muscles in the body (gluteals, hamstrings, and quadriceps) must be used continuously during the aerobic portion of the workout. According to these guidelines, a workout using only upper-body movements would not qualify as aerobic. The legs must be moving continuously for conditioning to occur.

Duration

The ACSM guidelines (regarding duration say that each workout should have a continuous aerobic portion, lasting between 20 and 60 minutes. Most exercise leaders consider 20 to 30 minutes the average for the aerobic portions of their classes. Classes with longer aerobic portions are usually of lower intensity and best for students who need to improve their body composition. Long-duration, low-intensity classes have shown to be excellent "fat burners." Programs with 30- to 60-minute aerobic portions are often called "calorie

burners." Longer duration, however, can also lead to overuse injuries. Students should gradually build up to longer aerobic sessions. The principle of progressive overload must be followed.

Intensity

The ACSM guidelines regarding intensity state that the exercise intensity of the aerobic portion should be in a range of 50% to 85% of maximum oxygen uptake or maximum heartrate reserve, or 60% to 90% of maximum heartrate. Beginning students should work at a low intensity and a low duration until adaptation begins to occur. Only people in excellent physical condition should work at an intensity in the upper portion of the range.

Frequency

The ACSM guidelines regarding frequency state that the workout should occur three to five times a week in order for results to occur. Working out fewer than three times a week does not assist in improving cardiorespiratory fitness levels. Working out more frequently than five times a week can prevent the body from rebuilding and cause overuse injuries.

Cooldown

The cooldown usually lasts about five minutes and uses large, lower-intensity, rhythmical movements. The purpose of the cooldown is to aid in returning blood to the heart at a low enough intensity to allow the heart to move toward a resting level. The cooldown prevents the pooling of blood in the extremities, reduces muscle soreness, and assists in the elimination of metabolic wastes.

The cooldown in the pool is especially important because of the pressure of the water. If a participant exits the pool while still in the aerobic portion of the workout, dizziness can occur. When exercising at a challenging intensity the blood vessels dilate to allow for the increase in bloodflow during the workout. When exiting the pool, the lessened effect of air pressure compared to water pressure allows the blood vessels to dilate further, causing the blood pressure to drop. This can cause the participant to feel lightheaded or dizzy or to actually pass out.

Toning

If toning or calisthenics are included in the workout they usually follow the cooldown. Trunk, upper-body, and lower-body exercises are done at pool edge or with buoyant devices holding the participant off the bottom of the pool.

Muscular Endurance

Some exercisers work on muscular endurance with many repetitions, and others work on muscular strength with fewer than 15 repetitions. If muscular strength is desired, students should be able to fatigue the muscle in fewer than 15 repetitions. The same exercises can be used for endurance and strength, but the level of overload and therefore difficulty has to increase. Exercise difficulty can be increased by using a larger range of motion, slower repetitions, more difficult exercise modifications, or aquatic exercise equipment. Students should provide force in each move to challenge the muscles and keep the body at a comfortable temperature.

Muscular Strength

If strength training is used during the toning portion, it should follow the ACSM guidelines for resistance training. Strength training of moderate intensity, sufficient to develop and maintain fat-free weight, should be an integral part of an adult fitness program. The recommended minimum is one set of 8 to 12 repetitions of 8 to 10 exercises that condition the major muscle groups at least 2 days per week.

The toning portion of the workout can last 5 to 15 minutes. Upper-body toning is often incorporated into the cooldown to conserve time. Because of the buoyancy of the water, participants must be strongly encouraged to put forth the necessary effort to make water exercise effective. It is very easy to cheat during water exercise because of the buoyancy and the relaxing effects of the water.

Flexibility

The water aerobics class should always end with a poststretch or flexibility section that lasts about five minutes. If the water is warm (over 86 degrees), this section can be extended. All the major muscles used or toned during the workout should be stretched during this time.

ACSM's revised Position Stand of 1998 recommends, "Flexibility exercises should be incorporated into the overall fitness program sufficient to develop and maintain range of motion. These exercises should stretch the major muscle groups and be performed a minimum of two to three days per week. Stretching should include appropriate static and/or dynamic techniques."

The purpose of the poststretch is to provide long-term flexibility, help prevent muscle soreness, lower the oxygen demands on the heart further, and reestablish the body's equilibrium. Each muscle should be stretched beyond its normal resting length to the point of tension but not pain.

Some aquatic exercise programs combine the toning and flexibility portions of the class to keep the student's body temperature comfortable and to be sure that the muscles being stretched are warm and pliable. After doing toning exercises for the hamstrings, participants would stretch the hamstrings. Following toning of the abductors, students would stretch the abductors.

Types of Aquatic Exercise Programs

Water Walking

Definition

Water walking is simply striding in waist- to chest-deep water at a pace fast enough to create the overload necessary for cardiorespiratory benefits. The type of stride used should be varied to ensure use of all the major muscle groups in the lower body. Most frequently, the foot action involves a heel strike followed by rolling onto the ball of the foot and finishing with a strong push off the toes. Stride length will vary according to the participants height, leg length, strength, and stride as well as the water depth. The type of walking—for instance forward, sideways, or backward with toes pointed in or out; with legs straight or bent; or moving on toes or heels—will all vary the muscles being used. Upper-body muscles should also be varied by using stroke, backstroke, figure eight's, punching, and jogging arms. Walking sideways usually offers less resistance and can be less exertive. Arm and directional variations can also vary the intensity.

Diagram 4-1   Water Walking

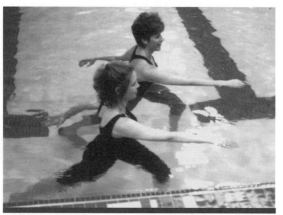

Format

The program should follow the format for an aerobic-conditioning class, beginning with a thermal warm-up, prestretch and cardiorespiratory warm-up, followed by the aerobic portion, the cooldown, toning, and poststretch.

Equipment

Most water walkers use no equipment, but wearing webbed gloves and resistant leg equipment will make the walk more challenging. Walkers can also add variety by using buoyant leg equipment and by using different resistant, weighted, or buoyant pieces of upper-body equipment on different strides or laps.

Water Depth

Walkers usually begin in hip- to waist-depth water and walk to armpit depth before returning to shallower water. Some lucky walkers have the same depth during the entire route. Shallow water (hip to waist depth) is easier to walk in, and the pace will be faster. Deep water (midriff to shoulder depth) is more difficult to walk in and the pace will be slower. Using the same tempo for shallow and deep walkers will generally not work. Along the same lines, using the same music for shallow and deep walkers will not be effective. Deep water (midriff to shoulder depth) is better suited to water jogging (see the following section).

Common Errors

The two most frequent mistakes made in water walking are (1) leaning forward while walking and (2) using the same stride for the majority of the walk.

Proper body alignment is essential and should be thought of during the entire walk. The head should be held in a neutral position with the chin centered, the eyes should look straight ahead (not up or down), the shoulders should be back and relaxed, the rib cage should be lifted, and the abdominals should be pulled in with the buttocks tucked under (pelvic tilt). If viewed from the side, the walker's ear, shoulder, and hip should be aligned. Walkers who lean forward are probably trying to go too fast and can compromise the low back. Maintaining good body alignment will also improve abdominal and back muscle strength. Walking strides should be slow and controlled. The exception to the upright alignment is race walking in the water. Race walkers lean forward slightly. Race walking is not recommended for the general population. Participants should always use proper alignment, as described above, with the abdominals tightened and buttocks tucked to protect the low back.

The second error—using the same stride for most of the workout—will encourage muscle imbalance. Many walkers use their usual walking stride in the water. However, the normal walking stride contributes to overly tight hip flexors. Varying the stride will allow participants to offset the natural muscle imbalance everyone has. By simply backing up, participants can ensure the use of the hip flexors opposing muscle group, the gluteals. Changing to other strides will allow adductors, abductors, hamstrings, and quadriceps to have equal use. Walkers should use different stride variations that involve different major muscle groups to ensure muscle balance. Each stride should be used for an equal amount of time, unless a specific alternative plan has been set up.

Arm variations are also important. The pectoral muscles are usually tight, so using the trapezius and rhomboids against the water resistance is important. Triceps should be used to offset their imbalance with the biceps.

Water walkers need to be sure the pool bottom is comfortable for their feet.

Shallow-Water Jogging
Definition
Shallow-water jogging is much like water walking but is done with bounding or leaping steps. Participants who jog in the water are pushing up and partially out of the water and bouncing as they move through the water, as opposed to walkers who are striding with no bounce. Like water walkers, joggers also vary the stride by moving backward, forward, and sideways with heels kicking up behind, knees high in front, knees out to the sides, legs straight, or jogging on toes or heels. Long, slow strides should be varied with short, fast strides. Arm movements should also be varied to provide upper-body muscle balance using backstroke, stroke, side push, punching, and jogging arms.

Format
The water-jogging program should follow the format for an aerobic-conditioning class, beginning with a thermal warm-up, prestretch, and cardiorespiratory warm-up, followed by the aerobic portion, the cooldown, toning, and poststretch.

Equipment
Water joggers need no equipment but can vary the intensity of the workout by adding lightly resistant or weighted upper-body equipment such

Diagram 4-2   Water Jogging

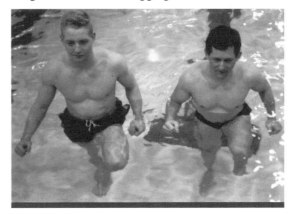

as webbed gloves or one-half- to one-pound wrist weights. Well-conditioned participants can jog with buoyant bells, heavier weights, or highly resistant equipment. Light ankle weights can be used and will not interfere with the stride but may offset some of the buoyant benefits of water jogging. If the purpose for water jogging is prevention or recuperation from injury, adding ankle weights is not recommended. Adding resistant or buoyant equipment may interfere with the stride for most participants. Well-coordinated, highly conditioned athletes may be able to use buoyant or resistant equipment on their legs.

Some water joggers need to wear special aquatic shoes to protect their feet from the bottom of the pool. The shoes will increase drag, which will in turn increase the intensity of the workout, but they will also prevent blisters, cushion the feet, prevent slipping, and help to absorb the shock of impact. Joggers may want to wear aquatic shoes or running shoes. Shoes with black soles may leave marks on the pool bottom. Joggers should be sure to wear white-soled shoes or shoes with nonmarking soles.

A tether is another piece of equipment that water joggers may need. If the pool being used is too small, joggers will become bored with changing direction so frequently. Using a tether system will keep the jogger in place while s/he still expends energy to meet the cardiorespiratory requirements. The tether system involves tubing that attaches to the edge of the pool or the stair or ladder rail. The participant wears a belt around his or her waist which attaches to the tubing. The runner tries to move forward but the tether keeps him or her stationary. Students must wear shoes to protect the bottoms of their feet.

Water Depth

Water jogging can be stressful to the joints if done in water shallower than waist level. The apparent weight loss of 90% in shoulder-depth water is reduced to about 50% at waist depth. The

impact of bare feet on a concrete or tile pool bottom at this depth can cause stress fractures and other overuse injuries. Midriff to shoulder depth seems to work best for shallow-water joggers. Some joggers wear buoyant belts and jog into the deeper end of the pool (5 to 12 feet) before returning to the shallow end.

Most shallow-water joggers prefer to keep their arms in the water to increase the resistance for upper-body toning, endurance, and workout intensity. Using arms out of the water and overhead can destabilize the body while moving through the water and cause alignment concerns.

Common Errors

Water joggers make three common mistakes: (1) jogging on the toes, (2) using the same stride for the bulk of the workout, and (3) leaning forward. On land, jogging is a heel-strike sport with the heel usually landing first. In the water, jogging is often done with the forefoot landing first. Too often, the participant never follows through to bring the rest of the foot down. Jogging on the toes can lead to general muscle soreness (torn tissue), tightness and shortness in the calf muscle, shin splints (a pain in the front of the shin), and if done in water too shallow, stress fractures (broken bones in the foot) or other overuse injuries. The jogger should always press the heel down to the pool bottom before pushing off again.

The second mistake—using the same stride for the major part of the workout—can lead to severe muscle imbalance and injury. Many joggers use their usual jogging stride in the water. However, the normal jogging stride contributes to overly tight hip flexors. Varying the stride will allow participants to offset the natural muscle imbalance everyone has. By simply backing up, participants can ensure the use of the hip flexors' opposing muscle group, the gluteals. Changing to other strides will allow adductors, abductors, hamstrings, and quadriceps to have equal use. Joggers should use different stride variations that involve different major muscle groups to ensure muscle balance. Each stride should be used for an equal amount of time, unless a specific alternative plan has been set up.

Arm variations are also important. The pectoral muscles are usually tight, so using the trapezius and rhomboids against the water resistance is important. Triceps should be used to offset their imbalance with the biceps.

The third problem—leaning forward while jogging forward through the water—is often a sign of trying to move too fast and can compromise the low back. Maintaining good body alignment will also improve abdominal and back-muscle strength.

Proper body alignment is always essential and should be thought of during the entire workout. The head should be held in a neutral position with the chin centered, the eyes should look straight ahead (not up or down), the shoulders should be back and relaxed, the rib cage should be lifted, and the abdominals pulled in with the buttocks tucked slightly under (a partial pelvic tilt). If viewed from the side, the jogger's ear, shoulder, and hip should be aligned. Joggers who lean forward are probably trying to go too fast and can compromise the low back. Most jogging strides should be slow and controlled.

Water Aerobics

Definition

Water aerobics includes a wide variety of dance and calisthenic moves done in the water. Water aerobics can be a very basic program, with extensive repetitions of kicks, jogs, and kneelifts, or it can be a highly choreographed program, combining intricate dance moves with calisthenic moves.

Format

Water aerobics classes usually begin with a

Diagram 4-3   Water Aerobics

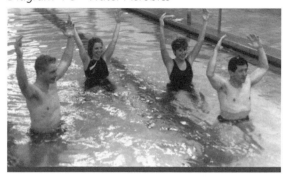

warm-up lasting 5 to 10 minutes. The warm-up portion begins with a thermal warm-up included to get blood and oxygen moving to the muscles and synovial fluid released in the joints. During the thermal warm-up, all major muscle groups can be involved in isolation exercises and low- to moderate-intensity exercises. Beginning with short levers and limiting the movement's range of motion is encouraged.

A prestretch segment is the next part of the warm-up. Stretches for muscle groups that may be tight from everyday living can be included here. Gastrocnemius (calf), iliopsoas (hip flexor), and pectoral (chest) muscles can all be considered tight muscles. Other stretches could include hamstrings (back of thigh), quadriceps (front of thigh), and spinae erector (low back). The prestretch is designed to lessen the likelihood of injury during the upcoming workout. It's important to keep the body temperature at a comfortable level during the stretches. If participants become chilled, muscles will contract and injury may result if stretching is continued. Keeping the upper body moving during lower-body stretches and vice versa can help to keep the muscles warm and pliable.

The cardiorespiratory warm-up is the last portion of the warm-up and includes increased range of motion and more moderate-intensity exercises. The purpose of the cardiorespiratory warm-up is to gradually increase the oxygen demands on the heart.

The aerobic portion of the workout uses the large-body muscles (quadriceps, hamstrings, and gluteals) continually with other major muscle groups to create the overload necessary to achieve cardiorespiratory fitness. This portion of the workout should last at least 20 minutes.

The cooldown usually lasts about five minutes and uses large, lower-intensity, rhythmical movements. The purpose of the cooldown is to aid in returning blood to the heart at a low enough intensity to allow the heart to move toward a resting level. If toning or calisthenics are included in the workout, they usually follow the cooldown. Trunk, upper-body, and lower-body exercises are done at pool edge or with buoyant devices holding the participant off the bottom of the pool.

The water aerobics class should always end with a poststretch or flexibility section that lasts about five minutes. If the water is warm (over 86 degrees), this section can be extended. All the major muscles used or toned during the workout should be stretched during this time. The purpose of the poststretch is to provide long-term flexibility, help prevent muscle soreness, lower the oxygen demands on the heart further, and reestablish the body's equilibrium. If participants become chilled during the poststretch, they can get out of the pool and stretch on the deck.

Equipment

Equipment is not necessary for water aerobics. The resistance of the water, the positioning of the limbs and body, and the force of the movements can all be used to increase the intensity of the aerobics program. The intensity can be further increased by using equipment designed for the fast and often shorter moves included in aerobics. Light wrist or ankle weight; moderately resistant webbed gloves, paddles, or footwear; and moderately buoyant ankle cuffs can all be used by the conditioned participant.

Water Depth

Midriff to armpit depth seems to be ideal for water aerobics. Participants will experience enough buoyancy to benefit from the lessened impact, and the arms will be partially immersed for upper-body toning benefits. Most participants are able to control each move at this depth. Shallower water could lead to stress fractures and other overuse injuries. Due to the lessened buoyancy in shallower water, there is increased impact and likelihood of injury. Shallow water also doesn't afford the chance for complete upper-body toning, since the arms are not immersed deep enough. Deeper water, while providing more buoyancy, does not allow the exerciser to fully control the exercise movements. Lack of control can lead to injury.

Common Errors

Water aerobics done in shallow water (hip to waist) can cause overuse injuries and possibly heat stress syndromes. When working out in shallow water, the participant should wear well-cushioned shoes or eliminate most of the bouncing from the program. To provide a safe, muscle-balanced workout, the program should incorporate a mixture of slow, full-range-of-motion moves and faster moves. All the major muscle groups should be used. Fast, ballistic moves can cause injury and should be eliminated from the program. A general rule to check on the safety of the speed of the move is control: If the move is controlled and the rest of the body is stable and aligned, the speed is usually safe.

Water Toning
Definition

Water-toning programs are created specifically to improve muscular endurance. Students work a specific muscle group with one move for 15 to 60 repetitions and then move onto another muscle group. Upper-body and lower-body exercises are usually alternated, with middle-body or trunk (obliques and abdominals) exercises interspersed throughout. Students usually stand at the pool edge or are supported by buoyant devices during the class.

Format

Water-toning participants must remember to include the thermal warm-up, prestretch, and poststretch portions of the program. (Review the preceding section on Water Aerobics for the content of each portion of the program.) The muscles and joints must be prepared for the work they will do during the workout.

The format for a water-toning program should begin with the thermal warm-up and prestretch which should last at least five minutes. If participants are not feeling warmed up at that point, the warm-up should continue until they feel comfortable in the water.

The toning portion of the class should follow the prestretch and can last anywhere from 15 to 40 minutes. Intensity in toning or endurance programs is determined by the amount of resistance used. Duration refers to the number of repetitions (reps) of each move performed within a time period and the number of times each group of reps is performed (sets). In general, toning or muscle-endurance training requires an overload in the number of repetitions. According to the rule of specificity, when designing a program for endurance development, low resistance and high repetitions should be used for maximum effectiveness. According to the principle of progressive overload, the instructor must progressively increase the overload on the muscle as it adapts to each new load. Frequency refers to the number of times an activity is repeated in a week.

A three- to five-minute cooldown with low-intensity, fluid, walking-level movements, followed by a poststretch of at least five minutes will finish the workout. Stretches during the prestretch only need to be held 10 seconds. Post stretches should be held 30 seconds.

Equipment

Most water-toning classes encourage students to use upper- and lower-body equipment after they have adapted to the water exercises without equipment. Webbed gloves, paddles, buoyant bells, small buoyant balls, and wrist weights can all be used to work the upper body. Balls, kickboards, buoyant bells, and resistant devices can all be used for middle-body work. Buoyant, weighted, and resistant ankle cuffs or boots can be worn to work the lower body. Stretchy exercise bands can also be used for lower-body toning.

Water Depth

Since students usually stand at the pool edge for water toning, midriff depth seems best. Participants are able to stand flat on the supporting leg and keep the body stabilized while doing lower-body exercises with the other leg. At this depth, participants will also be able to bend the knees slightly to immerse the entire muscle group being

Diagram 4-4   Water Toning

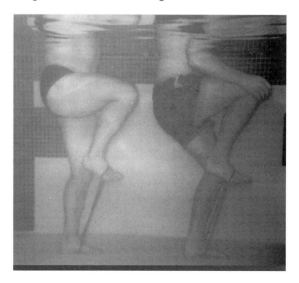

used during upper-body toning. Some classes use buoyant devices (kickboards, noodles, body buoys, deep-water vests or belts, etc.) during portions of the workout. Because of the amount of buoyancy the devices afford, many students are able to stay in midriff-depth water during the buoyant portion of the class. Others may have to move to deeper water at that time to keep their feet from touching the pool bottom during the exercises.

Common Errors

All the exercises must be controlled and done correctly. A general rule to check on the safety of the speed of the move is control: If the move is controlled and the rest of the body is stable and aligned, the speed is usually safe.

It is not a good idea to "go for the burn" during this type of exercise. Many water toners will experience the burn when they begin a program. After a few weeks, as the body adapts, the burn should occur less frequently. The burn is a sign of built up lactic acid. The exerciser should stop the move that is causing the burn and jog in the water for 20 to 40 seconds until the muscle gets the oxygen it needs and the sensation dissipates.

Strength Training

Definition

Strength training in the water is a program aimed specifically at body building. Actual weight-lifting moves, such as squats, bicep curls, knee extensions, and elbow presses, are done in the pool during this workout. In order to attain muscular balance and reduce the risk of injuries, all major muscle groups should be strengthened during a workout, including quadriceps, hamstrings, low back, abdominals, chest, upper back, shoulders, biceps, and triceps. Working all major muscle groups is important for a comprehensive and safe workout. Training just some of the muscles will provide less significant results, encourage muscle

imbalance, and could cause muscle injuries.

Format

A strength-training program begins with a thermal warm-up and prestretch. Since this is not a cardiorespiratory workout, no cardiorespiratory warm-up is necessary. The strength-training moves immediately follow the prestretch. Each muscle group that is strengthened during the workout must be stretched later. This final flexibility stage can be done either at the end of the workout or after the last set in which the muscle group is used.

Use Slow and Controlled Moves with a Minimum of Momentum It is important to perform the strength-training moves in a slow and controlled manner. Fast movements could place too much stress on the muscles, connective tissues, and joints. Fast strength training is less effective and more dangerous than slow strength training. Participants will be able to work with more resistance if they move quickly through the movements, but it will be momentum, not muscles, doing the work. Slow training uses more muscle tension, more muscle force, and more muscle recruitment and will be safer and more effective.

Diagram 4-5   Strength Training

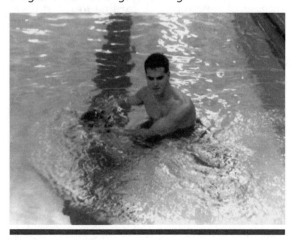

Full Muscle Extension to Complete Muscle Contraction Full range of motion movements should be used in strength training. This will ensure not only a full muscle contraction but also will allow the opposing muscle to stretch. Using a short range of motion will have limited value on the muscle being strengthened and could lead to a reduction in joint mobility. To test for full-range-of-motion in a joint, contract the muscle and move the joint without resistive equipment. When equipment is added, the joint should be able to move to full flexion and stop just short of full extension.

Systematic, Gradual Progression. The principle of progressive overload is extremely important in strength training. The resistance and repetitions should be gradually increased. The training stimulus must gradually overload in order to allow the muscles, bones, connective tissues, and joints to adapt without injury. Workouts that are more demanding require more recovery time so progression and frequency must be carefully crafted.

Equipment

Some unconditioned people are able to do strength training in the water without equipment. Highly conditioned athletes will require some type of resistance equipment.

Hydro-Tone and Aqua Fins are both types of resistant equipment used for upper-, middle-, and lower-body exercises. Participants should never hold their breath while using resistance equipment. Exhale during the exertive lift or press, and inhale during the return or rest portion. The equipment should be gripped easily, since a clenched grip can increase blood pressure.

Almost all strength training in the water is done with equipment based on the principle of resistance. Buoyant equipment does not work as well because only one muscle of each muscle pair will strengthen from the buoyancy offered. Weighted equipment that has been approved for use in the water is not heavy enough to create the overload needed to achieve strength benefits.

Water Depth

Strength trainers usually stand in water of midriff to armpit depth. Lower-body exercises are usually done standing at pool edge. Participants are able to stand flat on the supporting leg and keep the body stabilized while doing exercises with the other leg. At this depth, they will also be able to bend the knees slightly to immerse the entire muscle group being used during upper-body exercises.

Diagram 4-6   Strength Training

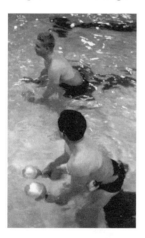

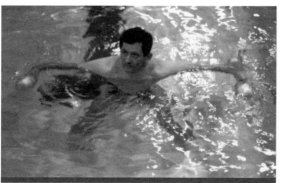

Common Errors

Injuries common to weight lifters can occur in the water if students begin with too much resistance or too large a range of motion or if they move too fast. All the exercises must be controlled and done correctly. A general rule to check on the safety of the speed of the move is control: If the move is controlled and the rest of the body is stable and aligned, the speed is usually safe. Correct form is vital. When muscles are too fatigued to maintain correct form, the exercise should be stopped.

Without actual weight in the water, strength trainers may slow down and in effect reduce the weight they're training with as they tire. The participant must be continually conscious of supplying maximum effort. Some students enjoy working with a metronome or with music at a specified beats per minute to keep them from slowing down.

Participants should maintain the natural curve of the spine and keep feet parallel, knees soft, abdominals contracted, chest open, shoulders down and slightly back, and the back of the neck open. Instructors and students alike will be able to watch for postural imbalances by using these hints for good form. Hyperextension of the lumbar area of the spine, hip flexors, knees, and elbows should be avoided.

Strength-training program participants must remember to include the thermal warm-up, prestretch and poststretch portions of the program. The muscles and joints must be warmed, lubricated, and prepared for the work they will do. The intensity in strength training will be determined by the amount of resistance that is used in the water. The duration refers to the number of repetitions (reps) performed of each move within a specific time period and the number of times each group of repetitions is performed (sets). In general, strength training requires an overload in the amount of resistance.

According to the rule of specificity, when designing a program for strength development, high resistance and low repetitions should be used for maximum effectiveness. Frequency refers to the number of times per week the activity is performed. All muscle groups that are strengthened should be stretched at the end of the workout or at the end of the use of that muscle group.

Guidelines

In early 1990, the ACSM set specific guidelines for resistance training programs. Those guidelines state that the frequency should be at least two times a week; this is considered a minimum standard and should be increased as conditioning occurs. It generally takes 48 hours for the body to repair and rebuild itself to a greater level of strength after a strength-training workout. Workouts, therefore, should be equally spaced throughout the week. Taking too little time between workouts can cause the workouts to be counterproductive.

The ACSM duration guidelines recommend a minimum of 8 to 10 different exercises during the workout. Each exercise should be performed at least 8 to 12 times (repetitions). This would be one set. While one set is the minimum considered for training to occur, more conditioned students should do multiple sets. Most muscles should be adequately stressed with 60 to 90 seconds of continuous contraction against a heavy resistance. That usually converts to 8 to 12 repetitions.

Flexibility Training

Definition

Flexibilty-training participants stretch different muscle groups to improve their long-term flexibility. Flexibility is an often ignored component of fitness.

If a muscle is only trained to contract, it loses its ability to stretch as far as it should, resulting in permanently shortened muscles. Most aquatic-fitness programs, such as toning, aerobics, and weight training, concentrate only on training the muscles to contract. Each aquatics program should include a flexibility segment.

Participants are often confused between the terms muscle and joint when attempting to understand how a flexibility class works. Muscles are elastic, which means they can stretch and have the ability to return to their normal position. Muscles that are tight, either from activities of daily life or from overuse in an exercise class, will shorten the range of motion in the joints they move. Increased range of motion in all joints is the goal of a flexibility class. The goal is achieved by stretching the muscles that move the joints. The joint is not stretched, the muscle is. The stretched muscle, in turn, increases flexibility and therefore range of motion in the joint.

Muscles that are tight from activities of daily living will need special attention during a flexibility program. Most of the population is round shouldered (scapula protraction) and need to stretch the pectorals. Tight hip flexors and gastrocnemius will also need special attention during the program.

Format

During a flexibility-training class, students

Diagram 4-7   Flexibility Training

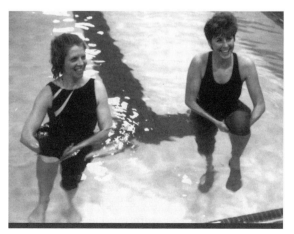

warm up a muscle group by using it and then move into a 30- to 60-second stretch of that muscle group. For example, students may do knee extensions for 30 to 60 seconds followed by a 30- to 60-second stretch of the quadriceps. Hamstrings would be worked next with knee flexion and then stretched. Intensity is determined by overload or the amount of lengthening occurring in the muscle beyond its resting length. The duration is determined by the type of stretching being done, how long each stretch is done, and how often each stretch is used. A frequency of three times per week is recommended for flexibility training. Care must be taken in flexibility training not to overload in ways that are harmful to the body. Muscles, like taffy, are much more pliable when they are warm. Muscle temperature is greatly affected by the water temperature. If muscles are used and warmed before stretching, safer stretching will occur.

Only static, never ballistic, stretches should be used. Fast, jerky, bouncing (ballistic) stretches can cause injury to the tendon and microscopic tears to the muscle tissue. Muscles are protected by a stretch-reflex mechanism. When a stretch is begun, a nerve reflex sends a message through the brain to the muscle fibers to contract. If a ballistic stretch is used, the muscles will be contracted when the next bounce occurs. Attempting to stretch a contracted muscle can cause injury.

Static stretches also cause the stretch-reflex mechanism to respond, but the static stretch will overcome the mechanism and allow flexibility to occur. The muscle fibers will contract at the beginning of the stretch, but if the stretch is held at that point (and not pushed further), the nerve will send the signal through the brain to have the muscle fibers relax again. When that occurs, the stretch can be taken a little further before the stretch-reflex responds again. Using the stretch-reflex concept in the program will help to increase flexibility gains. Participants should move to the point of mild tension and then relax as they hold the stretch in that position. After about 10 to 15 seconds, they can increase the stretch by a fraction of an inch until they feel mild tension again and then relax as they hold the stretch in that position. If the tension does not decrease, the participant should ease off the stretch and hold it at that point.

Equipment

Most flexibility students require no equipment. The edge of the pool and sometimes a bar just below the water surface can be used during this kind of class. Some participants use buoyant devices, such as kickboards, pull buoys, buoyant ankle cuffs or boots and bells, to assist in holding the joint in a full-range-of-motion stretch. This is not recommended for the unconditioned or beginning student.

Water Depth

Average pool depth for the flexibility class is midriff level. Students should immerse joints with problems (stiff joints, areas recovering from injury or surgery, hot joints, etc.) during the warming and stretching segments. Flexibility classes can also use the deep end of the pool if students wear buoyant belts. Flexibility programs are usually offered in water over 86 degrees.

Common Errors

The two most frequent mistakes in water-flexibility classes are (1) stretching cold muscles and (2) stretching too far. When concentrating on flexibility, many students ignore or minimize warming the muscle before beginning to stretch it. If that happens, injury may occur. Cold muscles should not be stretched. Warming the muscle brings blood and oxygen to it and makes it pliable. Warming also allows synovial fluid to lubricate the joint that the muscles move. This will allow a more comfortable, larger range of motion stretch.

Too often, students feel that they should stretch until it hurts. The phrase most frequently used to describe a proper stretch is "move to the point of tension, never pain." If performed correctly, a stretch will elongate the muscle to a length greater than its resting length. Students should feel the stretch but never feel uncomfortable. Overall flexibility will be improved with proper stretching.

Sport-Specific and Sports-Conditioning Workouts

Definition

Sport-specific workouts are aerobic workouts that are designed to assist sports enthusiasts in developing the muscle strength and flexibility, skills, agility, balance, coordination and visual acuity needed in their sport.

Format

The format of the workout begins with the traditional thermal warm-up, stretch, and cardiorespiratory warm-up. Power, balance, coordination, and sports skills and patterns are worked on during the aerobic portion. The concept of interval training can be used during the aerobic portion of the workout. Strength conditioning or muscle endurance can be worked on following the cooldown. Flexibility for specific needs follows the strength-conditioning or muscular endurance portion.

Sport-specific conditioning can be done for enthusiasts in most sports: baseball, javelin, biking, running, downhill skiing, tennis, weight lifting, football, soccer, cross-country skiing, and track and field. Enthusiasts from different sports can all take part in the same class if different stations are used and time is spent with each participant before enrolling. The entire class would stay together during the warm-up and for some of the agility, coordination, and speed drills in the aerobic portion of the class to assure muscle balance in the workout. Participants would then move around the pool from station to station, each of which is designed to assist athletes in developing the skills and strength needed in their particular sports. If equipment were needed, it would be at pool edge at the station.

Following the specific exercises, the class would come together again for the cooldown, upper- and lower-body strength exercises (once again for muscle balance), and the flexibility segment. If sport-specific flexibility were necessary, it would follow the group flexibility segment and be done at stations also.

Equipment

The actual equipment that is used in the sport can be used in the pool. Baseball bats, golf clubs, and tennis racquets are seen in pools during sport-specific workouts. It is important to note that the equipment, like any aquatic equipment, should always be used with control and safety in mind. Aquatic equipment like Hydro-Fit, Aqua Fins, Hydro-Tone, Aquatoner, AquaFlex fitness paddles, and Spri tubing and bands are also used in sport-specific training to help to stretch, strengthen, and tone specific muscles. It is also used to help to simulate moves in the sport.

Water Depth

Water depth is often dictated by the type of sport a participant is training for. Runners and soccer players may want to improve conditioning in deep water. Baseball players, tennis players, and golfers will need to be in water deep enough to be sure that their swing or stroke can be accomplished underwater. Speed drills are usually started in shallow water (hip to waist depth) and moved deeper (midriff to armpit) as the workout progresses. Agility and coordination drills work well in midriff to armpit depth if they're for the upper body. Baseball drills for co-ordination, balance, and agility in fielding a

ground ball, and turning and throwing obviously work best in shallower water.

Diagram 4-8   Sport Specific and Sports Conditioning

Sport Specific

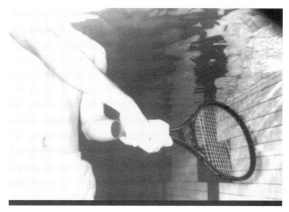

Sport Conditioning

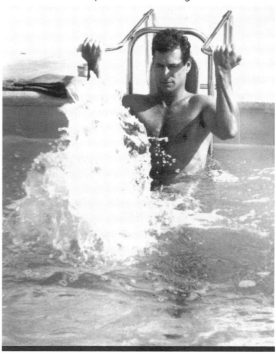

Common Errors

The mistake most commonly made in sport-specific training is to work on strengthening only those muscles needed during the sport. A goal in this type of program should be to assist in creating muscle balance in the athlete. All major muscle groups should be used. Determine the major muscle groups used in the sport, and strengthen those muscles overall. Develop agonists and antagonists equally.

Flexibility is too often ignored, even though it's importance in injury prevention has been well documented. All major muscles should be stretched, with special attention given to those muscles that need to stretch during the sport.

Sport-specific classes are usually designed for fit or conditioned participants who want to increase their abilities in their chosen sports. They are generally not classes for beginners or unconditioned individuals.

Interval Training

Definition

Interval training is an exertive exercise program usually reserved for well-conditioned athletes. The program can, however, be modified for less-conditioned populations. Interval training simply means a workout that combines high-intensity portions with moderate- or low-intensity segments.

During continuous aerobic training, the exercise program is organized so the workout intensity remains in the target zone during the entire workout. The intensity begins at the low end of the target zone and gradually increases to moderate and high intensity before tapering back down to the low end. Interval training is unique in that it is based on short bouts of intense exercise, during which the workout intensity is at the top end of the target zone. These high-intensity bouts are separated by recovery periods, during which the

workout intensity is at the low to moderate portions of the target zone. This technique trains the athlete to maintain near-maximum heartrate for a longer total time than would be possible with continuous training. This type of training uses the anaerobic metabolic pathway. The primary fuel is intramuscular glycogen.

Format

Intervals are usually done as the aerobics portion of a workout. The format for a cardiorespiratory workout is followed with a thermal warm-up,

Diagram 4-9   Interval Training

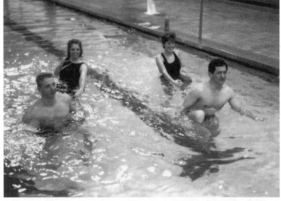

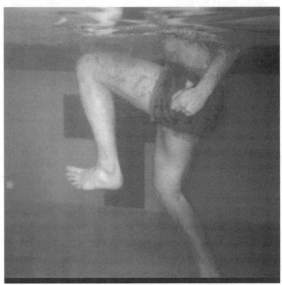

prestretch, and cardiorespiratory warm-up. The aerobics portion usually begins with three minutes of aerobics at low or moderate intensity. Approximately 75 seconds are allotted for the high-intensity interval before returning to moderate or low intensity for three more minutes. Five to seven cycles are done during the aerobics part of the program before cooling down, toning, and stretching.

A cycle is the combination of one low- (or moderate-) and one high-intensity set. The low- to moderate-intensity portion is usually at 60% to 75% of the target heart-rate. The high-intensity part of the cycle is usually at 75% to 80% of the target heartrate zone and is designed to move at least to and often beyond the anaerobic threshold.

The work-to-recovery ratio is how long the high intensity (work) lasts in comparison to the moderate or low intensity (recovery). Most interval-training programs use a 1 to 3 or a 1.5 to 3 work-to-recovery ratio. This means 60 to 75 seconds of high intensity (anaerobic) followed by three minutes of low to moderate intensity (aerobic) for each cycle. Some programs use a 1 to 2 ratio and others a 1 to 1 ratio. The most common is a 1 to 3 work-to-recovery ratio.

Equipment

Equipment is generally not used in interval training, unless it is part of a regular program for the recovery portion of intervals. For example, if gloves are usually used in the three-minute portion of the cycle, they can be left on during the high-intensity portion. In order to achieve the intensity required, aquatic equipment can be used if it can be added to the workout without interrupting or stopping it.

Water Depth

Water depth for interval training can vary, depending on the type of training being done. Since the concept of intervals can be used in deep-water running, water walking, or water aerobics, all different levels can be used. The depth commonly used for the regular program (water walking, aerobics, deep-water running) is the depth that should be used when intervals are added.

Common Errors

Instructors leading interval-training classes need to be aware that increasing the speed of the movements might elevate the heartrate and perceived exertion level but may compromise the joints and connective tissues. Too many times, instructors try to increase the intensity by only increasing the speed of the movements. Using equipment, increasing frontal resistance, increasing acceleration, and using long levers can all increase the workout's intensity. Moving through the water will also increase the energy requirements.

Interval training, like all fitness programs, should work toward improving participants' muscle balance. All major muscle groups should be worked and stretched during the workout.

Modifications can be made to the program to allow less-conditioned individuals to participate. The 3-minute moderate-intensity portion can be followed by a 75-second low-intensity portion, while other participants are doing 75 seconds of high intensity. The 75-second part of the cycle can be the recovery for less-conditioned participants.

Deep-Water Exercise

Definition

Deep-water exercise refers to any type of water exercise program done in the diving well of the pool or in water depth above the participant's head. It is a completely nonimpact workout. With every footfall on land, the legs bear two to five times the body weight; in deep water, the legs bear none.

Deep-water exercise usually falls into one of two

Diagram 4-10 Deep Water Training

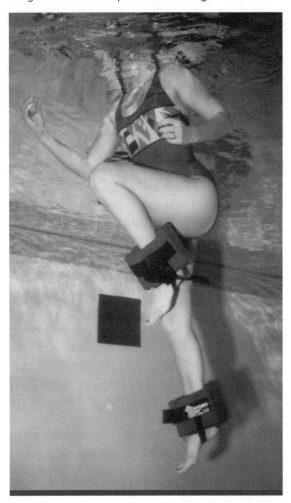

categories: running or exercises. Deep-water running is simply running, using different strides, in deep water. Deep-water exercises usually constitutes a class that follows the format for an aerobic workout, usually including some deep-water running. Deep-water exercises can be added to any program for variety.

Format

While many people get into the pool and start running immediately, a well thought out program will take the runners through a complete warm-up segment before beginning and finish with cooldown and flexibility segments after the run. Deep-water exercise programs should always follow the format for a safe, effective cardiorespiratory workout. (The format is reviewed at the beginning of this chapter.)

Exercises done in the shallow end can be done in the deep water with one variation: All movements are usually bilateral. Rather than kick one leg forward, a deep-water exerciser should kick one leg forward while kicking the other back. Rather than kick one leg out to the side, the deep-water exerciser should match the movement with the other leg to the other side. In order to keep good balance and alignment in the deep water, every move needs to be balanced by an opposite move.

Equipment

All participants in deep-water exercise should use flotation belts or vests. An AquaJogger, Wet Vest, Aqua Sizer, and any foam belt can all work to keep the exerciser afloat. Even good swimmers and floaters should wear flotation devices so that they can concentrate on performing the exercises correctly, rather than on treading water.

The workout intensity can be increased by using equipment like Hydro-Fit that not only keeps the participants afloat but also increases the resistance. These kinds of equipment use the concepts of bouyancy and resistance, rather than just buoyancy. As with all equipment designed to increase intensity, the principle of progressive overload should be followed.

Water Depth

Although most deep-water training occurs in water 8 to 12 feet deep, shallower water can be used. With the proper buoyant equipment, exercisers can do deep-water training in water three to four inches less than their heights. For example, a 5-foot, 4-inch woman could deep-water train in water five feet deep.

Common Errors

The most common mistake in deep-water exercise is poor alignment. Most exercisers lean forward, backward, or to the side during different exercises. Poor alignment makes the exercises simpler to do but keeps the proper muscles from actually doing the work. Leaning forward while running through the water makes it easier to cover more space, more quickly. Keeping the body in an upright, vertical, aligned posture creates more frontal resistance and therefore increases the intensity. This keeps the body in good alignment during training, causes co-contraction in the abdominal and back muscles (which serves to strengthen them), and allows the muscles that are being used to work, contract and elongate as they should.

Circuit Training

Definition

Circuit training is an aerobic workout that combines strength training and aerobic conditioning. It uses the aerobic and anaerobic energy systems. Circuit training takes place during the aerobic portion of a cardiorespiratory workout. The program follows the format for all cardiorespiratory workouts defined earlier in this chapter. The complete warm-up (thermal, stretch, and cardio) is followed by a 20- to 40-minute circuit-training aerobic portion. Participants work one muscle group, usually with equipment, for 30 to 60 seconds, and then move to aerobics for 1 to 3 minutes. Following the aerobic interval, participants work another muscle group. This is continued until all major muscle groups have been used. The cooldown follows, with the poststretch or flexibility segment at the end.

Format

Strength circuits are usually set up in stations around the edge of the pool so students can move

Diagram 4-11 Circuit Training

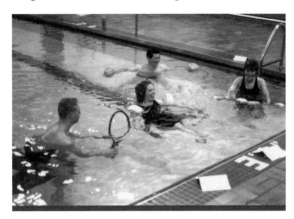

to a different station during each strength segment. This is called the self-guided method. Only students who are well motivated and understand how to perform the moves at each station will achieve good results. If participants need more help and there is enough equipment, everyone in the class can move to the edge of the pool and do the same strength move together. This allows the instructor to give the group motivational hints, correctional cues, and information on the muscle being used. This is called the group-travel method. People at all fitness levels are able to participate in circuit-training programs by personally modifying the intensity level of the strength and aerobic portions of the workout.

Equipment

Many different kinds of equipment can be used during circuit training. Tubing, bands, noodles or buoyant devices, resistant devices, and weights can all help to create the overload needed on the muscles during the strength circuits. The equipment should be simple to put on or be left on throughout the entire workout to be sure the training intensity level isn't lost.

Water Depth

Circuit training can be done at the shallow (midriff to armpit) end of the pool or in the diving well. If deep water is used, participants should wear flotation vests or belts.

Common Errors

A common mistake made during circuit training is to lose continuous movement and therefore aerobic training effect. Students who tire during the strength stations need to be reminded to keep moving even if they have to slow down. Students also can lose aerobic conditioning while moving to the pool edge if they don't move quickly. Picking up or putting on equipment is another time when students may stop continuous movement. If continuous movement isn't stressed, the workout will lose many of its benefits.

Strength-training moves should be full range of motion, slow, and controlled. All major muscles should be used during a circuit-training class. (Read the Strength Training segment, earlier in this chapter, for more information on speed of moves and muscle balance.)

Alignment is all important. Students' hips, shoulders, and ears should be in a straight line if viewed from the side. Proper postural alignment will help to prevent injuries in the exercise program.

The strength-training moves should be done with the idea of power and putting as much muscle as possible behind each repetition. Power, not speed, should be encouraged.

Plyometric Training

Definition

Plyometrics has become popular as a training technique to improve power, speed, and jumping abilities in athletes. Plyometrics involves a series of jumping, bounding, and hopping moves. The program begins with the easiest type of exercise (in place jumps) and progresses to the most demanding (bench jumps). Plyometrics is an anaerobic training program that is used by highly conditioned athletes whose sports involve power, speed, or jumping. It can be incorporated into a water aerobics class for the well conditioned. Plyometric moves work well in sport-specific-training, circuit-training, and interval-training programs.

In place jumps that can be used in plyometrics include scissor jumps, jumping-jack jumps, and tuck jumps. In place jumps begin with two feet and progress to one-foot jumps.

Hops are the next progression and include skipping, hopping, and hopping up steps. Participants begin in place and gradually move forward, backward, and sideways. During these hops, the athlete jumps up with complete plantar flexion of the ankle joint.

Bounding is the next progression. It involves both in place jumps and hopping but doing them to cover as much distance as possible.

Bench jumps are the final progression. These involve jumping on and off benches that are 10 to 20 inches high (depending on the conditioning level of the participant) using tuck jumps, long jumps, and side jumps.

Format

Participants begin with about 12 repetitions of each jump and progress to about 20. A total of 100 jumps per workout for a beginning program and 300 jumps per workout for an advanced program is average. Maximum effort should be expended during each move. A rest period of one to two minutes between exercises is required.

Equipment

Equipment is unnecessary for beginning students but can be added as students progress. Resistant equipment that increases drag will enhance the intensity. Other equipment, like aqua gloves,

Diagram 4-12   Plyometrics

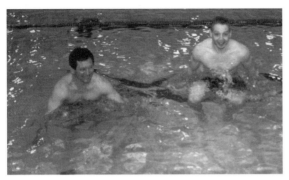

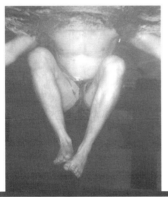

can improve distance jumps while using upper-body muscles.

Water Depth
Ideal water depth is midriff to armpit. Armpit depth is better for strong participants and those who cannot tolerate heavy impact. Waist to midriff depth is good for weak students if they can tolerate the impact.

Common Errors
The most common error made in classes using plyometric moves is to allow students to slow down and not use maximum effort. Participants should make an all-out effort all the time.

Relaxation Techniques
Purpose
Relaxation techniques are frequently used to augment or add variety to aquatic exercise classes. All of the techniques discussed can be done while in the water. It is possible to use just portions of any of these relaxation techniques during a two- to three-minute relaxation time at the end of class.

Participants will come to class unconsciously tense or tight because of stressful situations in their everyday lives. As the specific muscles that are tense or tight get tired of being continually contracted, they "give notice" by feeling sore and being stiff and by aching, freezing, or going into spasm. The muscles that are habitually contracted by tension are being forced to work when no work is required. This tends to shorten these muscles, which contributes to muscular imbalance, which in turn causes aches or pains and further tightening. Relaxation techniques can assist participants in improving muscle balance.

Types
There are two basic types of relaxation techniques. Muscle-to-mind approaches use muscular contraction and release to make the entire body—including the mind—relax. Mind-to-muscle techniques use the mind and its abilities to relax the entire body, including the muscles.

Muscles-to-Mind
Breath awareness is one example of a muscle-to-mind relaxation approach. Ai Chi is an example of this approach. Breathing techniques are the simplest tools for promoting relaxation. Simply being aware of each inhalation and exhalation begins the relaxation approach. Participants are encouraged to feel that fresh, clean air is entering the body during the inhalation and that impurities are leaving the body during exhalation. Participants are also asked to pay attention to the time between inhalation and exhalation; some count

Diagram 4-13   Relaxation

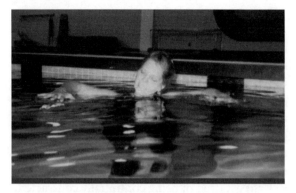

to any number between 4 and 10 during each inhalation and exhalation.

Progressive relaxation is another muscle-to-mind relaxation technique. Participants contract specific muscles in the body and then relax them to "let go." The progression generally goes up through the body, beginning with the feet; the progression can also work down, beginning with the head. Each muscle group is contracted approximately 5 times for 10 seconds each time. The first one or two contractions are strong all-out contractions. The following two contractions use only half the tension, and the last contraction is barely strong enough to be felt.

Mind-to-Muscle

Meditation is a form of mind-to-muscle relaxation technique. It focuses one's attention on a single syllable or sound. The participant attempts to totally clear his or her mind from any interfering thoughts or distractions.

Benson's relaxation response is another mind-to-muscle technique. A Harvard cardiologist named Herbert Benson brought some of the concepts and principles of Eastern forms of meditation to the West. His relaxation response technique is similar to meditation. The environment must be comfortable and quiet. Benson uses words such as "one" and "relax" as the syllable or sound to be

repeated. He recommends that participants have a passive attitude during meditation, allowing thoughts to come into the mind, gently pushing them back out, and refocusing on the word or sound.

Imagery or visualization is a relaxation technique frequently used by aerobics instructors. Ai Chi's bodymind approach allows it to fall into this category also. Research shows that by imagining themselves in successful situations, people can enhance their own success. This concept is used in imagery and visualization relaxation. The instructor often guides the class into a relaxing environment, such as a beach or mountain retreat. The relaxing environment is then described by the instructor in more detail, while the participants are able to relax as they visualize the new setting.

Autogenic training is a form of relaxation in which the body is trained to produce sensations of heaviness and warmth. The learning process is based on techniques similar to meditation and visualization, with the focus on concentration being the sensations. There are six stages of application for the technique:

1. heaviness in the arms and then the legs
2. warmth in the arms and the legs
3. heartrate regulation
4. breathing-rate regulation
5. warmth in the solar plexus
6. coolness in the forehead

Instructors using imagery and visualization talk students through this type of relaxation technique, going through each of the six stages gradually.

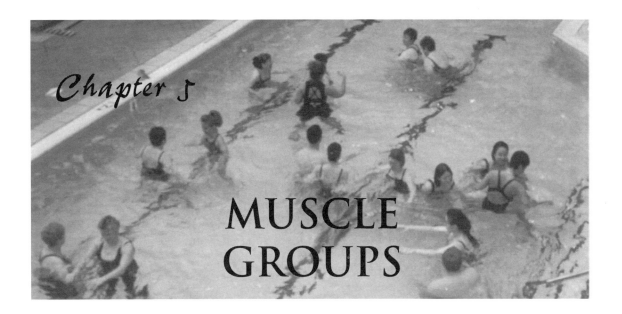

Chapter 5

MUSCLE GROUPS

Alignment & Muscle Balance

Good postural alignment allows the human body to move safely. From a front view, the shoulders should evenly align over the hip joints, and the pelvis should rest over the hip joints in a balanced position. From the side, the spine should have an anterior curve in the cervical and lumbar areas and a posterior curve in the thoracic area. The ear, shoulder, hip, and ankle joints should fall in line. When deviation from good postural alignment exists in one area, there is always a reactive deviation in another area.

Aquatic exercise instructors should not only teach proper postural alignment, but the exercises they teach should promote muscle balance. Muscles should be strong enough to contract fully when needed and to relax fully when contraction is not needed. Muscles that are hypertoned are unable to relax fully.

All the muscles surrounding each joint should be toned equally so there is a good balance and give and take among them. Each muscle should be of appropriate resting length, such that the bones and other body parts hang in proper neutral positions.

Muscles that are subjected to repeated overload will adapt by becoming stronger and wider. Unless they are specifically overloaded with a stretch, they will also become permanently tighter and shorter. When one muscle is consistently strengthened and the opposing muscle ignored, the strengthened muscle will become permanently shortened and the opposing or antagonistic muscle will remain lengthened, weak, and inefficient.

Muscle groups often work in pairs in order to first flex and then extend a part of the body at a joint. A good example of a flexor/extensor pair is the hamstring/quadricep muscle group. The hamstrings flex (bend) the knee, and the quadriceps straighten (extend) it.

Muscle balance is achieved when both muscles in a pair are developed to the same degree.

Imbalance, resulting from overdevelopment or underdevelopment of one member of the pair, can cause poor posture, pain, tendon tightness, and eventual misalignment of the body's framework.

Movements for Major Muscle Groups

The rest of this chapter outlines the major muscle groups. Each section ends with a list of toning, aerobic, arm, and stretch movements.

When designing a workout, the instructor should be sure to include at least two moves for each major muscle group in every hour-long program.

1. *Pectoralis/Trapezius/Rhomboids*

The pectorals are the chest muscles and cross the sterno-clavicular and shoulder joints. Their function is transverse adduction and medial rotation of the humorous. The pectorals are also responsible for depressing the shoulder girdle. The trapezius is a diamond-shaped muscle in the upper back and neck. It crosses the sterno-clavicular joint. The trapezius extends the head and neck and adducts and depresses the scapula. The rhomboids are small-back muscles located beneath the trapezius. They cross the sterno-clavicular joint and are responsible for adducting the scapula. The pectorals are the antagonists to the trapezius and rhomboids.

The exercises listed below will work the trapezius, rhomboids, and pectorals. When the arm movements go in front of or across the front of the body, they work the pectorals. When they move toward the sides and back, they work the trapezius and rhomboids.

> elbow press single
> elbow press with forearm down
> safe arms
> over and present
> scissor arms
> backstroke
> wind-up and present

Diagram 5-1   Pectorals

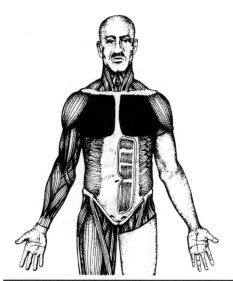

Diagram 5-2   Trapezius

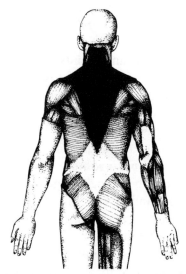

Muscle Groups

bow and arrow
reach pull in
stroke
waterpull
shoulder shrug
backstroke side

2. *Hamstrings/Quadriceps*

The hamstring muscles are located in the back of each thigh and cross the knee and hip joints. They are responsible for knee flexion and assist in hip extension and rotation. The hamstring's opposing muscle is the quadricep. The quadriceps are located in the front of each thigh and cross the knee joint. One of the quadriceps, the rectus femoris, also crosses the hip joint. The function of the quadriceps is knee extension and assistance in hip extension. The hamstrings are antagonistic to the quadriceps.

The exercises listed below will work the quadriceps and hamstrings: the hamstrings, as the knee is bent, and the quadriceps, as the knee is straightened.

jazzkick (also diagonal)
flick kick
jig
hoedown (also doubles, in 3)
hopscotch
heel hits behind
heel hits across
mule kick
ski bounce
paddlekick
forward lunge
Russian kick

3. *Biceps/Triceps*

The biceps are located on the front of each upper arm and cross the elbow and shoulder joints. The function of the biceps is to flex the elbow and assist in shoulder flexion. The opposing muscle is the tricep. The triceps are located on the back of each upper arm and cross the elbow and shoulder joints. The function of the triceps is elbow extension and assistance in shoulder extension.

Diagram 5-3   Quadriceps/Hamstrings

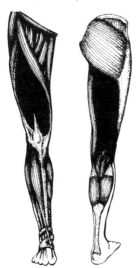

Diagram 5-4   Biceps/Triceps

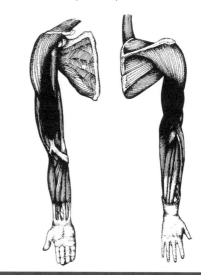

The exercises listed below will work the biceps and triceps. As the elbow bends, the biceps will contract. As the elbow straightens, the triceps will contract.

waist curl
tricep extensions back (also forward, out)
side press out, in
jog arms
lateral push
backstroke

4. *Iliopsoas/Gluteals*

The iliopsoas is a combination of two muscles: the illiacus and the psoas. Together, they are also frequently called the hip flexors. They are located on the front of the hip and cross the hip joint. Their primary function is hip flexion. They also flex the trunk. The opposing muscle is the gluteus maximus. It is located on the buttocks and crosses the hip joint. The function of the gluteus maximus is hip extension and lateral rotation of the hip joint.

The exercises listed below will work the iliopsoas when the hip flexes or the leg moves forward. As the leg comes back and lowers through the water, the gluteals will contract.

tuck jump
frog jump
kick
kick corner
kneelift (cross, out)
back kick (swing)
scissors (in 3, with back toes down)
knee swing
back lunge
leap forward
forward train
forward walking/jogging movements
flutter kick
scissor jump

Diagram 5-5   Iliopsoas/Gluteus Maximus

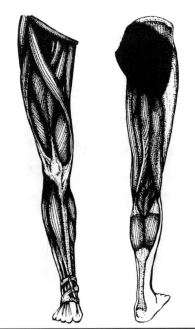

5. *Adductors/Abductors*

The adductors are located on each inner thigh. They cross the hip joint. The primary function of the adductors is hip adduction, or moving the hips together. The opposing muscle group is the abductors. The abductors are located on the outside of each thigh and cross the hip joint. Their primary function is hip abduction, or moving the hips apart.

The exercises listed below will work the hip adductors and abductors. As the limb moves laterally, the abductors will contract. As the limb returns to anatomical position, the adductors will contract.

crossing jog
side kick (forward and back, flex)
side circles
jumping jacks (doubles, in 3, crossing, jumps)

cross kick
heel hits front
fling
fling kick
kneeswing crossing
wringer
leap side
rock side
side train
side step

waterpull
twist
karate punch
press down and behind with sidebend
over and present
side scissors
rock side (in 3)
leap side
scissor turn
swing twist (in 3, move right and left, circle)
ski bounce

6. *Obliques*

The obliques are V-shaped and inverted V-shaped. They are located under and to the side of the rectus abdominus muscle. They cross the spine joints. The function of the obliques is trunk circumduction, lateral flexion and extension, and rotation. The obliques act as antagonists to each other.

The exercises listed below will work the obliques.

7. *Abdominals/Erector Spinae*

The erector spinae is a large back muscle that crosses the spine. Its function is head and spinal extension. The opposing muscles are the abdominals. The rectus abdominus is a large muscle that is located from the ribs to the pelvis and crosses the spine. The function of the rectus abdominus is spinal flexion.

There is a misconception that exercises that flex

Diagram 5-6   Adductors/Abductors

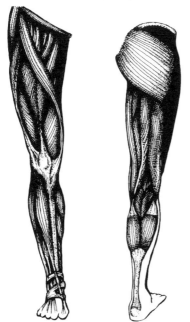

Diagram 5-7   Obliques

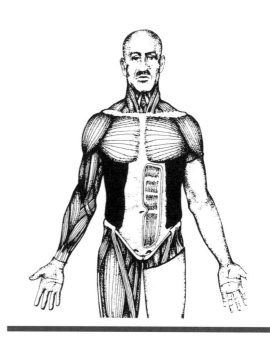

the hip are abdominal exercises. The rectus abdominus does not cross the hip joint and therefore is not the primary mover in hip flexion.

The exercises listed below will work the abdominals and back muscles.

> knees tucked crunch
> lift hips
> heel jack
> heel tilt
> pelvic tilt
> curl down
> jog tilt

8. *Anterior and Posterior Deltoids*

The anterior deltoids are located on the front of each shoulder and cross the shoulder joint. Their primary function is flexion and medial rotation of the shoulder joint. The posterior deltoids are located on the back of each shoulder and cross the shoulder joint. Their primary function is extension and lateral rotation of the shoulder joint.

The exercises listed below will work the anterior deltoids as the arm moves forward and the posterior deltoids as the arm moves backward.

> armswing, forward and backward
> with both elbows bent or straight arms
> swing forward and backward, alternating arms
>   forward and backward

9. *Deltoids (Medial)/Latissimus Dorsi*

The medial deltoid is a cap on the shoulder. It crosses the shoulder joint, and its primary function is to abduct (lift) the shoulder joint. The latissimus dorsi is a large back muscle in the middle on each side of the back. It crosses the shoulder joint, and its primary function is to adduct (lower) the shoulder joint. It also medially rotates and extends the shoulder joint. It depresses the shoulder girdle and assists in lateral trunk flexion.

The exercises listed below will work the medial

Diagram 5-8   Rectus Abdominus

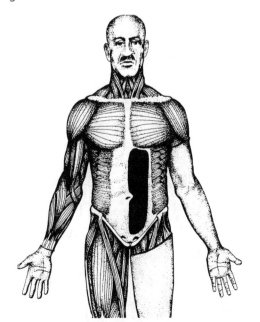

Diagram 5-9   Deltoids

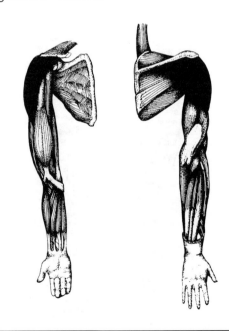

deltoid and latissimus dorsi. As the arms lift (ab-duct), the deltoid will contract. As they lower (ad-duct), the latissimus dorsi will contract.

press down behind
press down front
press down alternate
press down (one front, one back)
press down with elbows bent

10. *Gastrocnemius/Tibialis Anterior*

The gastrocnemius is located in the calf of each lower leg and crosses the ankle and knee joints. The primary function of the gastrocnemius is plantar-flexion. The tibialis anterior is located in the front of each lower leg and crosses the ankle joint. The primary function of the tibialis ante-rior is dorsiflexion.

The exercises listed below will work the gastroc-nemius as the toe points down (plantarflexes) and the tibialis anterior as the toe points up toward the shin (dorsiflexes).

bounce
most jogs
heel jack
heel tilt
scissor with front toe up
swing twist with toe up
kick and point, kick and flex

Diagram 5-10   Latissimus Dorsi

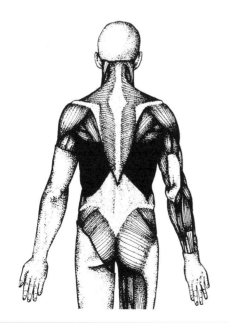

Diagram 5-11   Gastrocnemius

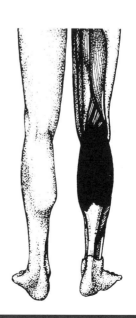

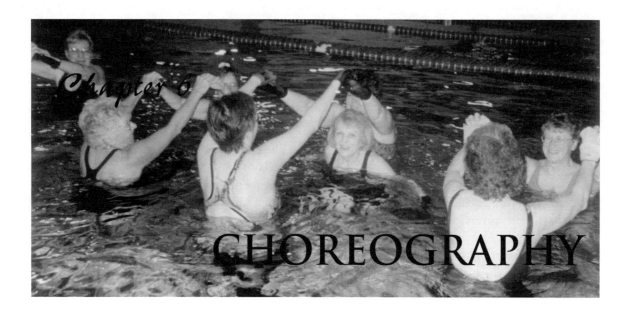

Chapter 6

CHOREOGRAPHY

Contraindicated Exercises

Aquatic exercise programs tend to have a large variety of populations and body types. For that reason, exercises that may be safe for one person may not be for another.

Some exercise is contraindicated which means that it is harmful to the exerciser's physical well-being. "Generally contraindicated" means that the exercise is contraindicated for the general population. "Relatively contraindicated" means that the exercise is contraindicated for some populations.

In order to create the safest possible program, the aquatic exercise instructor should be aware of two specific concepts when doing programming or choreography:

1. The purpose of each exercise—With this knowledge, the instructor can replace moves that may aggravate some students' conditions with other moves that have the same exercise purpose. For instance, a prone flutter kick primarily works the hip flexors (iliopsoas) and elevates the heartrate. Since prone flutter kicks have a high risk potential for low backs, an instructor could replace them with standing forward kicks, which have a lower risk potential but still work the hip flexors (iliopsoas) and elevate the heartrate. If the instructor then found that forward kicks were aggravating a student's low back, s/he could change the forward kicks to kneelifts, which also work the hip flexors and elevate the heartrate.

2. High-risk areas in the average body– The instructor must be aware of specific areas to protect, what those areas functions are, and what types of moves may compromise those areas. Instructors should use student's health history forms to determine specific vulnerabilities. When general high-risk areas for average populations and specific vulnerable areas in students are understood, the instructor can move on to beginning choreography. While moving through programming, the instructor should always compare the ratio of benefits of an exercise to its risk. If, in the instructor's point of view, the benefit outweighs the risk, s/he should use the move. There is the risk

associated with every type of move. Only those that seem to be high risk for the type of class should be eliminated.

High-Risk Areas

High-risk areas include the patellafemoral joint (knees), the shoulders, the cervical area of the spine (neck), the lumbar area of the spine (low back), and the ankle/foot.

Knees

The knees can be protected by remembering that their function is simple flexion and extension. Moves that are safe for the knee joint will not hyperextend it, twist the tibia in relation to the femur, move it too quickly, or overflex it.

Hyperextending the knees may occur during some toning moves but can also occur unintentionally during some aerobic exercises. For example, a forward kick, which should be safe for most populations, can become unsafe if students allow the knee to hyperextend as the leg returns from the kick. During the return, the hamstrings and gluteals need to contract to extend the hip joint. If the hamstrings and quadriceps do not also contract to tighten the knee joint into a slightly flexed position, the knee can hyperextend when it is pulled through the water resistance.

The instructor should analyze most exercise moves and educate the students to guard against knee hyperextension. Having students use "soft" knees (in a slightly flexed position) throughout the workout will help avoid this problem. Students should be aware, however, that "soft" does not mean there is not tension in the muscles surrounding the knee to protect it. Some instructors use the visual cue "move the leg as one unit" to give students the idea of tightening the quads and hamstrings.

Twisting of the tibia in relation to the femur causes torque in the knee. The knee is not meant to rotate when it is weight bearing or when participants are in a standing position. Twisting with the feet planted

can cause too much torque or twisting in the knee. A rule to follow to protect the knee joint from twisting is to keep the knee and toes of the same foot in the same longitudinal line (axis). This means that the knee and toes of one foot both point in the same direction at all times. If the knee points out, the toes also point out. If the knee points forward, the toes also point forward.

Twisting or torque can also occur during the return from a side leglift or sidekick when the adductors contract to pull the leg through the water back to anatomical position. The quadriceps and hamstrings should also contract to be sure the lower leg follows the upper leg without twisting the knee. If the quadriceps and hamstrings are not contracted, the lower leg can be twisted by the resistant forces of the water. The cross leg swing, described later in this chapter, can also cause twisting on the knee of the planted foot.

Movements should be slow and controlled when the knee joint is involved. Ballistic or percussive movements in the knee can cause injury. Extremely fast flexion and extension can cause damage to the joint capsule, tendons, and ligaments. Students sometimes use excessively fast movements during the toning portion at the end of class to enable them to feel the muscles working. Using force rather than speed during the toning will ensure a better and safer workout for the muscles.

The knees are not frequently overflexed in water exercise because the deep kneebends and squats that are frequently done in land-based exercises are almost impossible to do in the water. Overflexing of the knee is usually only a concern if the knee is weight bearing. In the water, participants may do deep forward lunges, which can cause the knee to overflex in a weight-bearing position. Forward lunges are safest if the knee of the forward foot is directly over the ankle. When the knee extends forward of the ankle and the foot, excessive stress is being placed on the knee joint.

Students sometimes have trouble feeling the

movement is large enough without overflexing the knee. If they are cautioned to take a larger step, the overflexion will usually not occur, and they will feel the movement has been large enough. Overflexing and possibly twisting the knee can also occur during quadricep stretches. The ankle and heel of the foot should be brought back only to the point that a stretch is felt in the quadricep or that there is no pain or discomfort in the knee. Some students will be able to pull the heel back to the buttocks with no pain in the knee. Others will have to stop part way into the flexion.

Shoulders

Shoulder impingement has become a concern of low-impact aerobic students and should thus also be a concern of aquatic exercise instructors and students. Seventy percent of the U.S. population has degenerative shoulder problems.

Shoulder impingement can occur in aquatic exercise when students spend a sustained period of time hanging from their arms on buoyant equipment or at the edge of the pool; maneuvering buoyant equipment and other weighted objects can have the same effect.

The shoulder joint is not made to support even the buoyant weight of a body in the water for very long. Exercises of this type should be done for only a short period before changing to another exercise that allows the shoulders to move back into their normal position.

When arms are abducted to shoulder position (90%), they should go no higher unless they are rotated into a supinated position and lifted the rest of the way.

Excessive and/or vigorous use of the arms overhead, as well as the use of weights with the arms overhead, can all increase the likelihood of shoulder impingement injuries. Using buoyant jugs that are partially filled with water as weights overhead is an extremely unstable move for the shoulder and should not be done.

Shoulder injury can also occur in the water when students move their arms from below the water surface to above the water surface. Moving arms in and out of the water needs to be controlled and occur near the body, rather than away from it. Doing jumping jacks with the hands at the sides and lifting them through the water, out of the water, and overhead can cause severe damage to the shoulders. At the beginning of the move, the deltoids contract to lift the arm against the water resistance. When the arm breaks free of the water, momentum rather than muscular contraction can take the arm past the safe range of motion. While lowering the arms, the deltoids eccentrically contract to resist the forces of gravity. As the arm hits the water, the latissimus dorsi have to suddenly contract to make the arm work through the water resistance. Shoulders can also be injured by lifting the arm forward through the water and allowing the arm to break the surface of the water.

Shoulder problems can be aggravated by a program that uses the joint with long levers before short levers. Warming up with simple shoulder rolls, adding the elbow, and then using the full arm would be a natural, progressive order. Beginning with the full arm as a lever may not allow the shoulder joint's synovial fluid and muscles enough warm-up to handle the long-lever stress without injury. Arm circles done out to the side with weights, resistant, or buoyant equipment can also cause shoulder injury.

Neck

The cervical vertebrae and discs can be injured during aquatic exercise. The cervical area of the spine has several functions, including flexion and extension, lateral flexion and extension, and rotation. It also is capable of hyperextension, which will be discussed later. A safe rule for aquatic exercise instructors is to allow the cervical area of the spine to move in only one of those functions at a time. This is a conservative way of viewing each of the moves the students do.

Instructors often ignore problems in the neck because their choreography does not include any moves for that area of the body. Unfortunately, students often involve the neck when doing other moves with the legs or arms. Instructors have to be extremely alert to watch for high-risk movements done in the cervical area of the spine.

Hyperextension of the cervical area of the spine should be eliminated from aquatic exercises. Students look up but not all the way up. Full-neck circles should be eliminated and replaced with a look down, a look somewhat up, a look to the right, then left, and a neck stretch (with the right ear to the right shoulder and then, the left ear to the left shoulder). Hyperextension can also occur during a prone flutter kick. Students will often hyperextend the cervical area of the spine when doing a backward-moving leg or arm exercise with force. During toning at the end of the class, students may hyperextend the cervical area of the spine when doing back kicks or kickswings-back to work the gluteals. Throwing the head back when the leg comes back compresses the discs of the spine and is a little like self-induced whiplash.

Percussive or ballistic moves in the cervical area of the spine can also damage the vertebrae and discs. Instructors would not purposely choreograph percussive neck moves, but doing fast kneelifts may make the students do fast neck flexion and extensions, too. Educating students on proper body alignment and constantly reminding them can alleviate this problem.

It is thought that one out of three people in the North American population has asymptomatic neck problems. With good visual cues and proper instruction, those problems need never become symptomatic.

Low Back

Eighty to ninety percent of the population in North America experiences back pain at some time in their lives. Low-back pain is the most common problem seen in our population. For that reason, exercises involving the low-back muscles should be well thought out.

The lumbar and thoracic areas of the spine have several functions. They can do spinal flexion and extension (bending forward and returning), lateral flexion and extension (sidebends to the side and returning), and rotation (twist). They can also hyperextend, which will be discussed later.

In terms of spinal flexion, lateral flexion, and rotation, a good rule is to allow the back to do only one of these functions at a time. If the spine is involved in forward flexion, it should not at the same time be involved in rotation. This sometimes occurs when students do crossing kneelifts. As the knee comes up and crosses, the spine rotates slightly. As the opposite elbow moves toward the knee, the spine continues to rotate. Problems occur when the student bends forward slightly to get the elbow all the way to the knee. Crossing kneelifts can be done safely by having the students keep their torsos tall and touch a wrist to the knee. This will still allow spinal rotation but eliminate spinal flexion at the same time.

Hyperextension of the lumbar area of the spine should be eliminated from all standing or moving exercises. Slight hyperextension during abdominal stretching should be the only exception to the rule of removing all arching or hyperextension of the low back throughout exercise. A 30-degree spinal hyperextension is okay to use for abdominal flexibility. Prone, facedown flutter kicks often create hyperextension in the low back. Changing the hand position at the pool edge will often alleviate the hyperextension of the lumbar area of the spine but will create hyperextension of the cervical area of the spine. Flutter kicks, if used at all, can be done slowly and with the face in the water.

While hip joints generally don't experience injuries themselves, extending the hip joint beyond five to ten degrees can radiate lumbar area hyperextension and cause low-back problems. The standing cross leg swing exercise (described later in this chapter) can cause back hyperextension and rotation at the same time. Extremely high forward kicks and cossack jumps can cause hyperextension of the lumbar area of the spine during the return to hip extension if they are done incorrectly. Toning double-leglifts, done with the back to the edge of the pool and elbows resting on the pool edge or with kickboards or a noodle under the elbows, can also cause back hyperextension during the return to hip extension.

Many of the exercises that compromise the low back are thought to work the abdominals, so students work them more vigorously and enthusiastically than they do other exercises. Very few abdominal exercises actually compromise the low back. The exercises that students and instructors think work the abdominals are actually working the iliopsoas or hip flexors. Instructors should be aware that if the spine (vertebrae) is flexing, the abdominals are working. If the hip joint is moving, the muscles working are the iliopsoas. Double-leg lifts and flutter kicks both work the iliopsoas. A safer way to work the iliopsoas is with standing forward kicks.

Hyperextension of the lumbar area of the spine may also occur as students move forward through the water. This is especially true if the legs are kicking backwards, as in back kick or mule kick, while the body is moving forward. While it is simpler to move forward with the legs kicking backward, it is safer and more intense to move forward through the water with the legs kicking forward.

Back kicks and sometimes mule kicks can also cause the low back to hyperextend. This happens for two different reasons: (1) Students try to kick back further than is necessary to work the gluteals or hamstrings (use only 5% to 10% hip extension) or (2) their arms move backward through the water at the same time the leg does. In order to relieve the strain in the low back from back kicks, the arms should move forward as the legs move backward.

Lateral flexion of the spine can also lead to injury if it is done in an unsafe manner. Students who do sidekicks during aerobics or side leglifts during toning at the side of the pool often try to lift the leg too

high. Hip abduction should only be done at 45 to 50 degrees. While the leg is abducting, the upper torso should stay straight up. Injuries can occur when students move out of proper alignment to do hip abduction. Lateral flexion can also cause a problem if it is done in a percussive manner. Waist bounces to the side can compromise the low back. Sidebends done with both arms overhead can also compromise the lumbar area of the spine.

All exercises involving the lumbar area of the spine should be slow and controlled. Ballistic or percussive moves can easily cause injury in the low-back area. While instructors would not intentionally choreograph fast spinal flexion and extension (bending forward and returning), students may incorporate it into moves themselves. Students often lean forward (spinal flexion) during kicks and kneelifts. They feel that their kicks or kneelifts are higher if they come closer to the chest.

Not only is this unwise in terms of maintaining proper body alignment, but it is especially unwise if the kneelifts are moving quickly and the students engage in percussive spinal flexion and extension. Sustained spinal flexion is not encouraged in any type of exercise for the general population.

Likewise, students sometimes find that walking or jogging through the water in a circle is easier if done leaning forward. It will involve more muscles and be more beneficial and injury free if it is done in an upright, vertical position. Slowing the tempo down or allowing students to move through the water at their own pace will allow them to maintain proper body alignment.

Instructors can assist students by teaching correct abdominal stabilization and pelvic mechanics. By contracting the abdominals and using them to hold the body in proper alignment, students can protect the low back through all exercises. It is mistakenly thought that back muscles are very strong and only need to be stretched. While it is true that they do need to be stretched, they are often not strong but simply tight. Isometric abdominal exercises for stabilization purposes can not only assist in firming abdominal muscles but in stretching the low back, too.

Lower Leg, Foot, and Ankle

The lower leg, foot, and ankle are susceptible to many overuse injuries. While these injuries are impressively lessened by working out in the water, they still can occur. Instructors should watch for students who have excessive pronation or supination. Many injuries are associated with students' specific anatomy. A person with excessive pronation (rolling in) of the foot is more likely to have an injury on the inside or medial side of the leg or ankle. Supinators, however, are more likely to have an injury on the outside or lateral portion of the lower leg or ankle.

Side-to-side movements of the leg seem to put additional stress on the foot, ankle, and lower leg. They do not need to be eliminated but simply done with control and stability. Many other ankle/foot injuries are caused by impact. The instructor can guard against this in three different ways: (1) moving students to deeper water; (2) adding a flotation belt or vest; and (3) creating a program with less bouncing and more walking or traveling moves. Too often, instructors feel the exercise intensity is best if all the moves are bouncing. Not only can exercise intensity be increased by striding through the water, it can also lessen impact injuries.

Impact injuries can also be lessened by teaching the students how to land. Students who stay on the forefoot can develop severe lower-leg and foot injuries. Having the students consciously think about landing first on the forefoot and rolling the heel down to the bottom of the pool and bending the knee can considerably lessen the likelihood of injury. Finding an adequate water depth for students and keeping the music tempo moderate enough to allow time to move in a controlled manner can lessen the likelihood of students twisting or spraining an ankle. Adding shoes that are designed for aquatic exercise can also help the instructor and student protect the foot and ankle. Shoes can also help the instructor

and student protect the bottoms of the feet from wearing an excessive amount of skin away and from slipping.

Repetitions

Excessive repetitions of one move that causes bouncing on the other leg can lead to an overuse injury and cause the support leg to become destabilized. It is prudent to bounce only eight times on one foot before changing to the other. Toning exercises where no bouncing on the other foot occurs can be repeated up to 30 or 40 times.

Traveling Moves

Lateral, forward, or backward, movement will increase the intensity of the workout. Traveling can also increase the risk of the workout. To minimize the risk, the instructor should caution students on proper alignment before beginning the traveling move.

Tempo

The speed, or tempo, of the exercise or music should allow enough time to move each exercise through a full range of motion in a controlled manner. Movements designed to go through a 50% range of motion should be allotted adequate time to complete that purpose. Percussive, ballistic, or jerky types of movements can cause injuries throughout the body. The water will soften many of these moves and students will subconsciously modify the moves for their own safety, but neither provision will be adequate for total safety. The instructor must maintain a speed of movement that will be appropriate for the type of program and student.

A Catalog of Movements

Moves are listed in alphabetical order for convenience. Major muscle groups involved are listed in the description of each movement. Many moves begin in one of the basic positions listed here.

Starting Positions

Feet Together – stand, with the feet lined up, neither foot forward of the other, and no more than six inches apart

Prone – lie on the water surface in a face-down position

Stride Position – stand, with the feet shoulder-width apart, toes and knees pointed forward

Supine – Lie on the water surface in a face-up position

Arm Movements

Suggested arm movements are often listed for step movements, and step movements are often listed with arm movements. Arm movements may use the following terms:

Corresponding or Opposite – Corresponding refers to movements in which the arm and leg on the same side of the body move together, in the same direction. Opposite refers to movements in which the arm on one side of the body moves in the same direction as the leg on the other side of the body.

Doubles and Singles – Doubles indicates that both arms move together with the same movement, in the same direction. Singles indicates that only one arm is doing the movement.

All the moves listed in this section of the book can be used with all types of choreography and in any type of program (i.e., deep water, interval training, aerobics, sports conditioning).

Individual Moves

– Abdominal Stretch

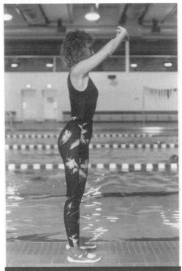

Abdominal Stretch
While standing, lift ribs and push your rib cage forward. This will cause a slight hyperextension of the lumbar area of the spine. Use with caution.

Abductor Stretch
While standing on one foot, pull the heel of the right foot toward the front of the hip of the left leg. Press the right knee in toward the left shoulder for the Abductor Stretch right. Reverse for Abductor Stretch left.

– Abductor Stretch

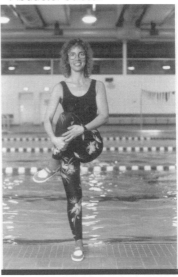

Choreography

Adductor Stretch

Take a big step to the left side with the toes of both feet pointed forward. Feet will be more than shoulder width apart. Bend the left knee but keep the right knee straight. This will stretch the adductors in the right leg. If the water is too deep for this stretch to be effective, lift the right knee up and to the right to stretch the right adductors. Reverse the above to stretch the left leg adductors.

Anterior Deltoid Stretch

See Bicep, Anterior Deltoid, and Pectoral Stretch.

Anterior Tibialis Stretch

See Iliopsoas Stretch.

Armswing Forward

Begin with arms down at sides with palms back (pronated). Lift both arms forward through the water with force until the arms are extended in front of the body just beneath the water surface. This portion of the move works the deltoids and pectorals. Keeping palms down, press both arms back to beginning position. This portion of the move works the deltoids and latissimus dorsi. Proper body alignment should be maintained during the Armswings. This move can be varied by alternately swinging one arm forward as the other swings back.

Armswing Forward Flexed

Begin with arms down at sides, elbows bent (flexed) at a 90 to 120 degree angle, and palms back (pronated). Lift both arms forward through the water while maintaining the original elbow flexion until the arms are in front of the body just beneath the water surface. This portion of the move works the deltoids, biceps and pectorals. Keeping the palms down, press both arms back to beginning position. This portion of the move works the deltoids, biceps and

– Adductor Stretch (version 1)

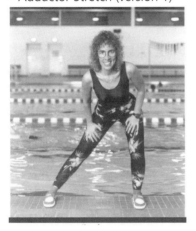

– Adductor Stretch (version 2)

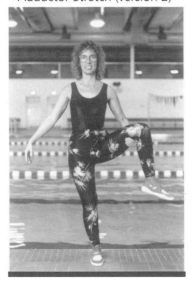

– Armswing Forward

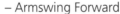
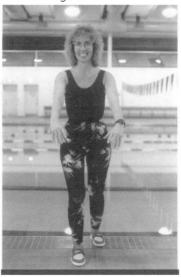

– Armswing Forward Flexed

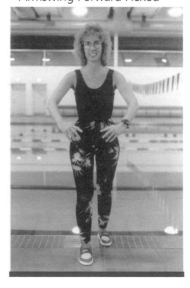

latissimus dorsi. This move can be varied by alternately swinging one arm forward and the other swings back.

Armswing Side

Begin with arms down at sides with palms back (pronated). Move both arms to the right and then up toward the water surface to the right. This is Armswing Right. Return arms to beginning position. Move both arms to the left and then up toward the water surface to the left. This is Armswing Left. Return arms to the beginning position. This move can be varied in several ways. Armswing Right with right arm only and Armswing Left with left arm only would be a Single (one arm only) Corresponding (the same side) Armswing right or left. The elbow can be slightly flexed to create variety. Palms can be pronated so hands slice through the water or they can push through the water with the backs of the hands leading or with the palms cupped and leading for added resistance. Armswings side work the deltoids, pectorals and trapezius.

Back Kick

Begin with feet in stride position and arms at sides. Without flexing (bending) the knee, kick the right leg back (hip hyperextension). Return to beginning position and repeat the movement with the left leg. To protect the low back, the right arm should swing forward, punch forward or elbow press when the right leg kicks back. Both arms can swing, punch or press forward when either leg kicks back. It is not advisable to move arms back when the leg is moving back since it may compromise the low back. Back kicks can be done slow with a bounce between each one or fast, kicking one out while the other is returning. Another variation is alternating the kicks right and left or done in groups of 2,4, or 8 right before changing to the left leg. Back kicks work the gluteals and iliopsoas.

Back Kick Swing

Begin with feet in stride position. Kick the right leg forward (hip flexion) for the first count and swing it straight back to slight hip hyperextension for the second count. The Back Kick Swing gives a larger range of motion while working the gluteals than the Back Kick. Abdominal muscles should be contracted while the leg is swinging back for back safety and the work should be felt in the gluteals. Back Kick Swing works the iliopsoas and gluteals. It can be done alternating right and left legs or done in groups of 2,4, or 8 with one leg before switching to the other. The left arm should swing forward as the right leg kicks forward, and the right arm should swing forward as the right leg swings back to avoid compromising the low back.

– Armswing Side

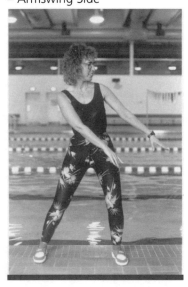

– Back Kick

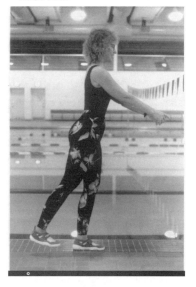

Back Lunge

Begin with feet in stride position and arms extended laterally (out to the sides) with palms facing forward. Step the right foot back and shift the body weight to the

– Back Kick Swing (position 1)

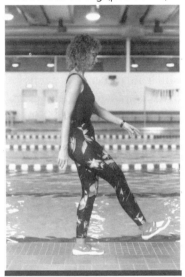

right foot while keeping the left foot down in beginning position. During the step back, arms move forward just beneath the water surface until palms almost meet. Return right foot to beginning position while pressing arms back to beginning position. Repeat with left foot. This move works the gluteals, iliopsoas, pectorals and trapezius.

Back Stretch

Begin facing the pool edge with the hands and arms extended over pool edge. Bring the knees to chest and hug knees. See also Erector Spinae.

Back Touch

See Touch Back.

Backstroke

Begin with both elbows in at

waist and forearms out to side for the short backstroke. With the palm supinated (facing forward) and elbow flexed and staying in at waist, reach back with the hand, cup the water and pull it forward (almost a complete circumduction of the elbow). This can be done alternating the right and left arms or it can be done using both of them together. The short backstroke works biceps and triceps. The long backstroke is the same move with arms extended. Both arms begin extended laterally with palms down just beneath the water surface. Reach back, turn the palm to face front, cup the water and pull it down and forward. This move works the deltoids, trapezius and pectorals and can be done alternating the right and left arms or doing both

– Back Kick Swing (position 2)

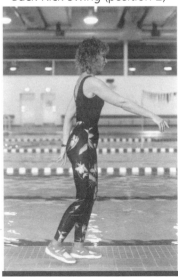

– Back Lunge

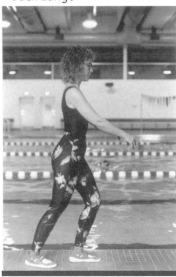

– Short Backstroke

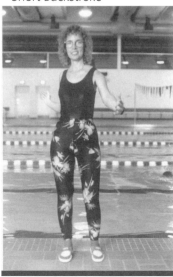

at one time. Both backstrokes are excellent moves for moving back through the water.

Backstroke Side
With the right arm extended just below the water surface back to the right (behind the body) with a slight flex in the elbow and palm facing the right, pull the right arm forward and left just below the water's surface until it is extended directly in front of the body. Return to beginning position and repeat with the left arm extended back to the left and moving forward. This move works pectorals, serratus anterior, deltoids, rhomboids and trapezius. Performing the same move using the forearm only (the action will be in the elbow not the shoulder) will work biceps and triceps. It can be per-

formed using both arms at once in either manner. It works well with any ordinarily stationary move either done in place or moving backwards.

Baseball Swing
Using both arms, swing back and then forward as though hitting a baseball. Repeat on the left side.

Basketball Jump
Bounce three times in a low crouched position while mimicking bouncing a basketball. Push up and out of the water as far as possible while mimicking shooting a basketball.

Bicep, Anterior Deltoid, and Pectoral Stretch
With fingers interlaced, low behind the back, turn elbows in toward each other and lift the arms up behind the back until a stretch is felt in the pectorals, anterior deltoids and biceps. Keep the chest out, chin in and back straight.

Bicep Curl
Begin with elbows in at waist and hands down with palms forward (supinated). Bend elbows (elbow flexion) to a 90 to 120 degree angle for the first count. Return to beginning position for the second count. This is one bicep curl. Bicep curls can be done singly by doing 8 to 16 with

– Long Backstroke

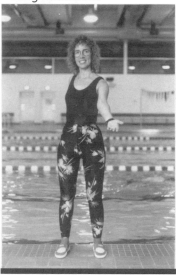

– Backstroke Side

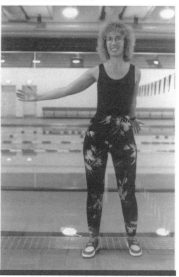

– Bicep, Anterior Deltoid, and Pectoral Stretch

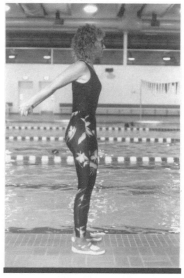

one arm before switching to the other arm. This is often done during toning. They can also be done alternating right and left arms. Bicep curls work the biceps.

Boogie

Begin with feet in stride position. Step the right foot behind and to the left of the left foot. The left foot remains stationary and the torso faces forward or may twist slightly while the exerciser looks to the left. The left arm reaches down to the left diagonal, while the right arm comes out of the water and reaches up to the right diagonal. This is the first count. Return to beginning position for the second count. The left foot steps behind and to the right of the right foot while the participant looks to the right and keeps the torso either facing forward or slightly twisted. The right arm reaches down to the right diagonal and the left arm comes out of the water to reach up to the left diagonal. This is the third count. Return to beginning position for the fourth count. These four counts represent one set of boogie. The boogie works obliques, adductors and gluteals. The boogie can be done four or eight times with the right foot before changing to the left. Arms can be varied to be kept beneath the water surface by using fly arms.

Bow and Arrow

Begin with both arms extended laterally (out to the side) to the left side at shoulder level. Feet, knees, hips and shoulders are pivoted to the left to allow the palms to begin together. With feet, knees and hips stationary, pull the right elbow back until right fist is near the right shoulder. To eliminate the oblique work for people with back problems, allow the feet, knees and

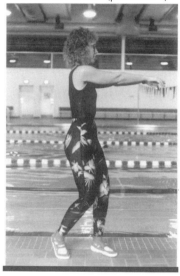

– Bow and Arrow (position 1)

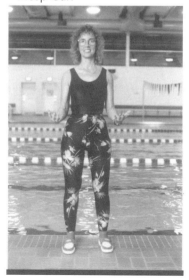

– Bicep Curl

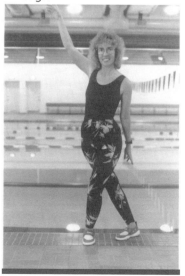

– Boogie

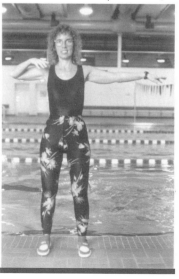

– Bow and Arrow (position 2)

hips to pivot with the shoulders. Continue with several repetitions using the right arm before switching to the left. Pectorals, deltoids, trapezius and rhomboids are all involved with this move.

Buffalo Shuffle

The buffalo shuffle moves laterally with four or eight buffalo shuffles moving to the right followed by four or eight buffalo shuffles returning to the left. Begin in stride position. Step the right foot laterally to the right with the knees, toes and torso facing forward and the left foot kicks out slightly to the left side. The right arm comes out of the water and points to the right diagonal while the left arm is on the left hip. This is the first count of the buffalo shuffle. The

left foot steps behind the right foot while the right knee comes up. The elbow of the right arm comes down to the water surface. This is the second count of the buffalo shuffle. Repeat counts one and two three or seven more times moving to the right. For buffalo shuffle left, step laterally to the left with the left foot while knees, toes and torso face forward and the right leg kicks out slightly to the right. The left arm comes out of the water and points to the left diagonal while the right hand is on the right hip. This is the first count of buffalo shuffle left. Step the right foot behind the left foot while the left knee comes up. The elbow of the left arm comes down to the water surface. This is the second count of buffalo shuffle left. Repeat

counts one and two of buffalo shuffle left three or seven more times to complete a set of buffalo shuffles. The buffalo shuffle works adductors and abductors.

Calf Stretch
See Gastrocnemius Stretch.

Cross Kick
Begin with feet in stride position with the right hip slightly rotated externally (right toes will be pointed to the right diagonal). Cross and lift the right heel in front and to the left of the left ankle. Return to beginning position. With the left hip slightly rotated externally (left toes will be pointed to the left diagonal) cross the left heel in front and to the right of the right ankle. Return to the beginning position. The Cross Kick works

– Buffalo Shuffle (position 1)

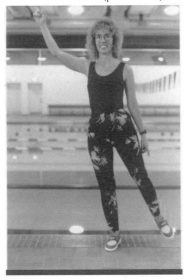

– Buffalo Shuffle (position 2)

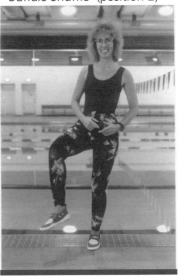

– Cross Kick

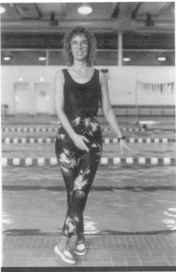

adductors and abductors. The move must be made with the heel leading through the water. If the hip rotates internally and the toes point to the opposite diagonal and lead the move, the iliopsoas will be involved. The torso should be kept facing forward during the Cross Kick. Lateral push to the right when the right leg is crossing to the left, and reverse.

Cross Rock

The cross rock is much like a rocking horse with the legs in a crossed position. Begin with the weight on the left foot and the right leg lifted (hip flexion) slightly across the left leg. Step the right foot forward and across the left foot, leaning the body forward toward the left (over the right foot) while keeping the

body straight. Avoid any spinal flexion that might cause the body to bend at the waist. The left foot will come up off the pool bottom and kick back slightly to the right as the weight is shifted to the right foot. This is the first count of Cross Rock. Step the left foot back to beginning position and lean the body slightly back to the right, while keeping the body straight. Avoid any spinal hyperextension that might cause the body to bend backwards at the waist. The right foot will come up off the pool bottom and kick forward to the left as the weight is shifted to the left leg. This is the second count of Cross Rock. Repeat counts one and two three more times and then switch to Cross Rock left, with the left foot rocking forward and across the

right foot and the right foot rocking back and to the left. The Cross Rock works iliopsoas, gluteals, obliques and abdominals. Safe arms, pushing back as the body leans or rocks forward and pushing forward as the body rocks back work well with this move. This move can be varied to Cross Rock Doubles as described in Rocking Horse Doubles, but crossing the rock. It can be varied to Cross Rock in Three, or Cross Rock Three and Doubles as described in Rocking Horse in Three but done with a cross. It can also be varied to Cross Rock Seven and Up as described in Rocking Horse Seven and Up but with a crossing rock.

Crossing Jog

The crossing jog moves laterally to the left in sets of four or eight and then returns to the right. Begin with feet in stride position and hands on hips. Cross the right foot over and toward the left of the left foot and shift the weight to the right foot while lifting the left foot slightly off the pool bottom for the first count. Step the left foot laterally to the left of the right foot and shift the weight to the left foot for the second count. Repeat counts one and two 3 or 7 more times while moving sideways through the water to the left. Reverse by crossing the left foot over the right and shifting the weight to

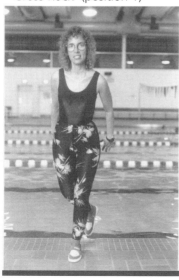

– Cross Rock (position 1)

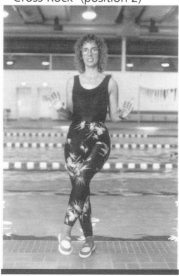

– Cross Rock (position 2)

the left foot for the first count. Step the right foot laterally to the right of the left foot and shift the weight to the right foot for the second count. Repeat counts one and two three or seven more times while moving right. Arms can stay on hips or can push laterally to the right when moving left and push laterally to the left when moving right. Keep the torso facing forward to achieve the excellent oblique, adductor and abductor work the Crossing Jog provides. The Crossing Jog can also be done with the leading foot crossing behind instead of in front as described above. While moving left, the right foot would step behind the left foot for the first count of each two count segment. While moving right, the left foot would step behind the right foot during the first count of each two count segment. This is called Crossing Jog Behind and also works the adductors and abductors. The Crossing Jog in front and behind can be combined to create a grapevine move. A two count segment of Crossing Jog in front moving left would be followed by a two count segment of Crossing Jog Behind moving left and repeated twice before reversing to move to the right. This can be called a Crossing Jog Combo or a Grapevine. The cues would be "cross, step, back, step, cross, step, back, step".

Crossing Legswing
Begin standing with back to pool edge. Lift the right leg (hip flexion) until it is at a 90 degree angle, with the knee slightly flexed (bent). Cross (horizontally adduct) the right leg toward the pool edge on the left side of the body for the first count. Return leg to beginning (forward) position for the second count. Swing it out (horizontally abduct) toward the pool edge on the right side of the body for the third count. Return it to beginning position for the fourth count. This is one Crossing Leg Swing. Repeat seven more times with the right leg before switching to the left leg for eight Crossing Leg Swings. The Crossing Leg Swing works the adductors and abductors. This move can severely compromise the stability of the weight-bearing knee. If this move is used, the weight bearing knee should be slightly flexed and never feel any twisting movement. The range of motion for the Crossing Leg

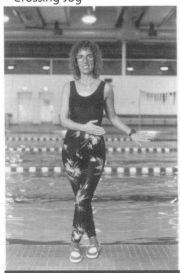
– Crossing Jog

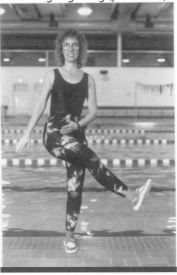
– Crossing Legswing (position 1)

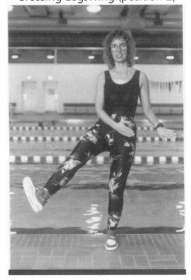
– Crossing Legswing (position 2)

Swing should be very small. The Knee Swing Crossing may be a better choice for adductor and abductor work.

Curl Down

Begin with arms extended (shoulder flexion) straight in front of the body just below the water surface. Bend forward (forward spinal flexion) at the waist bringing the sternum and navel closer together. Return to upright position. As the spine bends forward, keep the shoulders and elbows tight and the arms will be forced down deeper into the water. The arms themselves should not do the moving (avoid any shoulder extension) but only move because of the spinal flexion. The arms will create a drag, and force the abdominal muscles to work during the flexion. Students should be cautioned not to bend at the hips as this will work the already strong iliopsoas muscles. The bend or flexion should occur only at the waist. Holding a buoyant device (kick board, ball, etc.) in the hands will increase the difficulty of the abdominal work.

Crunch

Buoyant bells, balls or noodle needed. In a supine position (lying on back), flex knees and hips. Round shoulders forward and "crunch" shoulders to knees. Do not extend to straight leg position. Works the abdominal muscles.

Deltoid Lift

Begin with both arms down at sides with palms in at thighs (supinated). Lift the arms with force to the sides and up (abduct). This portion of the move focuses on the deltoids. To reverse the move, press both arms down through the water. This portion of the move works the latissimus dorsi.

Deltoid Stretch (Medial)

Begin with a neck stretch. When the head is tilted to the left side, reach behind the back with the left arm and pull gently on the right wrist. Reverse for deltoid stretch left.

Deltoid Stretch (Posterior)

With right arm at shoulder level, pull right elbow in toward chest with the left hand and bend the right elbow to feel the stretch in the posterior deltoids. Reverse for posterior deltoid stretch left.

– Curl Down

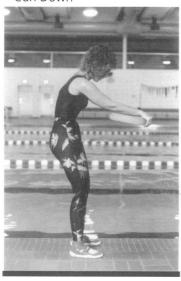

– Deltoid Lift

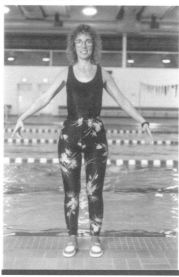

– Deltoid Stretch (Medial)

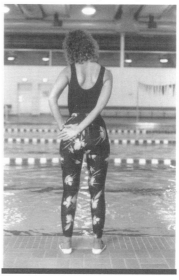

– Deltoid Stretch (Posterior)

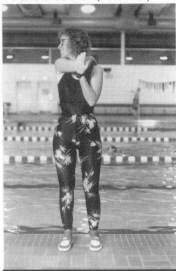

Diagonal Kick
See Kick Corner.

Elbow Press
Begin with both arms out to sides (extended laterally). Elbow is flexed to 90 degrees with forearm straight up from elbow. Lower arms into water. Begin the move in this position. Press elbows and hands toward each other (shoulder adduction) until they almost touch. Pull elbows and hands apart to return to the beginning of the move. The primary movers during the press are pectorals and serratus anterior, while the pull works the rhomboids and trapezius. Jogging, mule kicks and heel tilts all work well with these arms. Be sure arms are below water surface if possible.

Elbow Press Single
Begin in the position above. Press right elbow across body (shoulder adduction) to the left which has not moved. Stop and pull elbow back to beginning position (shoulder abduction). Repeat with right arm if desired and then repeat the press with left arm. Swing twists and bounce twists work well with these arms.

Elbow Press with Forearm Down
Begin with both arms out to sides (extended laterally). Elbow is flexed to a 90 to 120 degree angle with forearm straight down from elbow. This will cause forward (anterior) shoulder rotation in most people. Widen the angle until no shoulder stress is experienced. Begin the move in this position. Press elbows and hands back toward each other behind the back. This

– Elbow Press

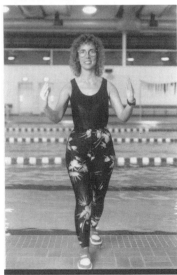

– Elbow Press Single

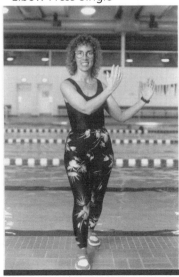

– Elbow Press with Forearm Down

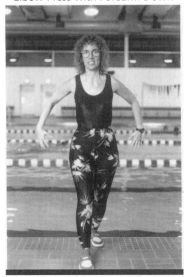

works the rhomboids and trapezius. Bring arms forward to return to beginning position.

Erector Spinae Stretch

With toes and knees pointed forward and feet shoulder width apart, put hands on the front of the thighs. Pull abdominals in and arch back up to feel the stretch. If the water is too deep, the stretch can be done with hands interlaced and pushing forward.

Flag Arms

Begin with hands on hips and elbows out to the sides. While keeping the right elbow in its position in space, lift the forearm forward and up until the forearm points straight up. The fingertips should be just beneath the water surface. This rotates the right shoulder externally. The left forearm moves down and back while the left elbow retains its place in space. The left forearm should be pointing straight down. This internally rotates the left shoulder. This is the first position of flag arms. Reverse by pressing the right forearm forward and down (internally rotating the shoulder) and lifting the forearm forward and straight up (externally rotating the left shoulder). This is the second position of flag arms. Repeat positions one and two to work shoulder rotator cuff, deltoids and trapezius.

Flick Kick

Begin with weight on left leg and right hip externally rotated (turned out). Right knee flexes and extends (bends and straightens) four times. This is flick kick-4. Repeat with the left leg. The flick kick works quadriceps and hamstrings. To increase the work on the quadriceps, move forward to the right

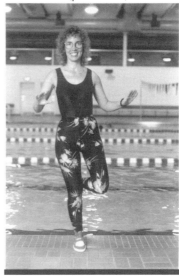
– Flick Kick (position 1)

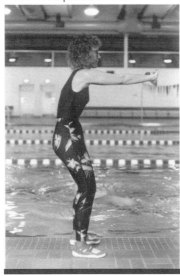
– Erector Spinae Stretch

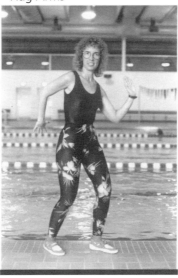
– Flag Arms

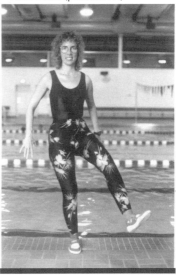
– Flick Kick (position 2)

or right diagonal during the flick kick right. To increase the work on the hamstrings, move back during the flick kick.

Fling

Begin with the weight on the left leg and the right hip externally rotated (turned out). Flex (bend) the right knee to about a 90 degree angle. Begin the move in this position. Lift the right heel forward as high as possible while maintaining the knee flexion, hip flexion and proper body alignment. The left (opposite) arm can come out of the water and reach overhead, or stay underwater and press from abduction (arm straight out to the side just beneath the water surface) toward the right heel. Step the right foot down and repeat with the left foot and right arm. The

Fling can be done "slow" with both feet bouncing together between each Fling or it can be done "fast" with the left heel lifting while the right one is returning and visa versa. The Fling can also be done in groups of 2, 4 or 8 right before switching to the left leg.

Fling Kick

Begin with weight on the left foot and the right hip externally rotated (turned out). Flex (bend) the right knee slightly. Begin the move in this position. Lift the right foot forward as high as possible while maintaining the knee flexion, hip rotation and proper body alignment. Step the right foot down and repeat with the left leg. This move is much like a Kick with the toes pointed out. To ensure

adductor work, the heel and instep should lead. The Fling Kick can be done "slow" with both feet bouncing together between each kick, or "fast" with the left foot moving forward while the right foot is returning. It can be done in groups of 2, 4 or 8 with the right leg before switching to the left leg. The Fling Kick works adductors and abductors. Refer to Fling for optional arms.

Flutter Kick

This move is usually done in a floating position with kickboards or other buoyant devices under the arms. It is also frequently done in a prone position (lying on the stomach) with hands on pool edge. With knees locked in slight flexion (bend), flex and extend (bend and straighten) the hip. The right leg kicks forward as the left leg kicks back and the left leg kicks forward as the right leg kicks back. This move works iliopsoas and gluteals. This move can compromise the low back (lumbar area of the spine) if done in a prone position with the face out of the water.

Forward Lunge

Begin in stride position with arms extended forward (shoulder flexion) and palms facing out (away from each other). Step the right foot forward and shift body weight to the right foot while bending the right

– Fling

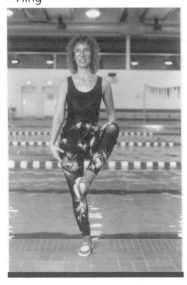

– Fling Kick

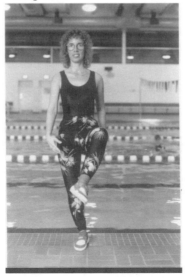

knee as the arms push straight back (as in Safe Arms). This is the first count. Step the right foot back to stride position as the arms return to beginning position. This is the second count. Repeat counts one and two with the left foot. This move works quadriceps, hamstrings, pectorals, rhomboids and trapezius.

Forward Touch
See Touch Forward.

Forward Train
Begin with feet in stride position with arms forward just beneath the water surface and palms back. Step the right foot forward and shift weight forward while bending the right knee and pushing arms back until they're extended laterally (out to the

sides). The left foot lifts off the pool bottom behind the left leg. This is the first count. Step left foot back into beginning position while the right knee lifts and arms return to beginning

position. This is the second count. Step right foot back and shift the body weight back on to the right foot while the left knee lifts and push arms forward and together for the third count.

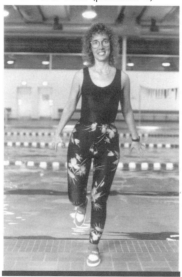
– Forward Train (position 1)

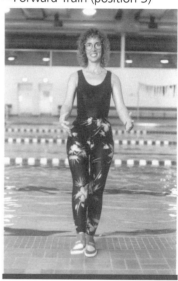
– Forward Train (position 3)

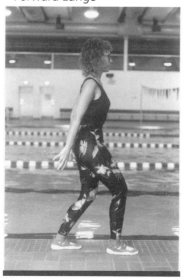
– Forward Lunge

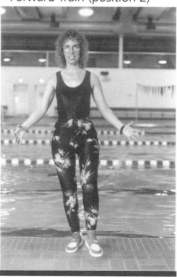
– Forward Train (position 2)

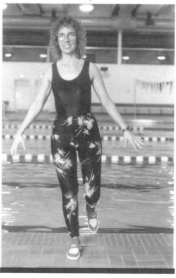
– Forward Train (position 4)

Step left foot forward to beginning position while the right knee lifts and arms return to the beginning position for the fourth count. This is one Forward Train with the right foot leading. Repeat three more times and then Forward Train four times with the left foot leading. Forward Train works pectorals, rhomboids, trapezius, iliopsoas and gluteals.

Frog Jump
Begin with feet in stride position with hips externally rotated (toes and knees pointed out). Pull both knees up toward shoulders. This is one Frog Jump. Push both arms down in front or press down behind during the frog jump. This move works the iliopsoas and gluteals. Maintain proper body alignment during the frog jumps.

Gastrocnemius Stretch
Take a big step forward with the left foot in front of the body and the right behind. Be sure the toes of the right foot are pointed forward or even slightly inward.

– Frog Jump

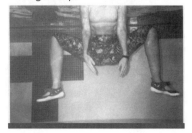

Heels must be down on both feet. Lean forward slowly and hold as the calf muscle of the back leg stretches. If the buoyancy of the water makes it difficult to feel this stretch, have the students think about pulling the toes of the back foot up. Reverse for gastrocnemius stretch left.

Gluteal Stretch
Pull the right knee toward the chest and hold it with hands under the knee (behind the thigh). Stand straight up on the left foot which should be pointed straight ahead with the knee slightly bent. Tighten the right knee as close to the chest as possible and hold. Reverse for left gluteal stretch.

Golfing
Use both arms to mimic a golf

– Gastrocnemius Stretch

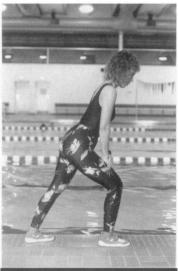

swing. Repeat on both the left and right side of the body.

Hamstring Stretch
Stand facing pool edge. Put the bottom of the right foot against the pool side or put the right heel into the pool gutter. Stand straight up. The left foot on the pool bottom should be pointed straight ahead with knee slightly bent. While looking straight ahead, bend forward at the waist and then straighten the right leg until a stretch is felt in the back of the thigh of the right leg. Reverse for the left leg. An alternative hamstring stretch is to begin in gluteal stretch position with the knee tucked close to the chest. While keeping the knee close to the chest, straighten (extend) the knee until an easy stretch is felt in the hamstrings.

– Gluteal Stretch

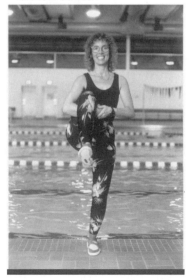

Heel Diamond

Buoyancy needed. In a supine position, place the insteps of the feet together. Keeping feet together flex knees and hips in lateral motion (pulling heels toward body) and return to normal semi-straightened position. Works adductors and abductors.

Heel Hit Out

Bounce once on the left foot while the right hand reaches back to touch the right heel as the right heel pulls up to the right of the right hip (knee flexion with internal hip rotation). Bounce once on the left foot while the right hand reaches back to touch the left heel as the left heel pulls up to the left of the left hip. The Heel Hits Across work the quadriceps and hamstrings. This move can com-

promise the knee joint. It is important to keep the torso tall and the spine straight during Heel Hits.

Heel Hit Behind

Bounce once on the left foot while the left hand reaches back to touch the right heel as it pulls up behind the left leg. Bounce once on the right foot while the right hand reaches back to touch the left heel as it pulls up behind the right leg. These Heel Hits work the hamstrings and quadriceps. It is important to maintain proper body alignment with a posterior pelvic tilt to avoid compromising the low back.

Heel Hit Front

Bounce once on the left foot while the left hand reaches down to touch the right heel as it pulls

up in front of the left thigh. Bounce once on the right foot while the right hand reaches down to touch the left heel as it pulls up in front of the right thigh. These Heel Hits work the adductors and abductors. It is important to keep the torso tall and spine straight during the Heel Hits.

Heel Jack

Begin with feet in stride position. Bounce once on the left foot while tilting slightly back to the left and touching the right heel forward to the right diagonal on the pool bottom. This is the first count. Bounce once with both feet together for the second count. Bounce once on the right foot while tilting slightly back to the right and touching the left heel forward to

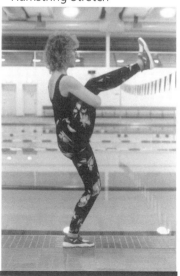

– Hamstring Stretch

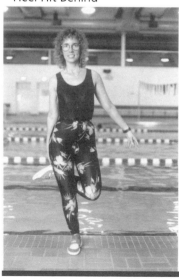

– Heel Hit Behind

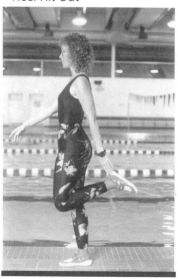

– Heel Hit Out

the left diagonal on the pool bottom. This is the third count. Bounce once with both feet together for the fourth count. This is one set of slow Heel Jacks. Arms can press down behind as the heel touches forward and out. The Heel Jacks work the abdominals, obliques and tibialis anterior. Heel Jacks fast can be done by leaving out the second and fourth counts. During the fast Heel Jacks the left arm punches through the water down toward the right foot while the right heel touches. The right arm punches through the water down toward the left foot while the left heel touches.

Heel Jack in Three

Begin with feet in stride position. Bounce once on the left foot while tilting slightly back to the left and touching the right heel forward to the right diagonal to the pool bottom. This is the first count. Bounce once with both feet together for the second count. Bounce once on the right foot while tilting slightly back to the right and touching the left heel forward to the left diagonal to the pool bottom. This is the third count. Bounce with both feet together once for the fourth count. Bounce once on the left foot while tilting slightly back to the left and touching the right heel forward to the right diagonal for the fifth count. Bounce both feet together once for the sixth count. Bounce once on the left foot while tilting slightly back to the left and touching the right heel forward to the right diago-

nal for the seventh count. Bounce both feet together once for the eighth count. Cue as: Right, Bounce, Left, Bounce, Right, Bounce, Right, Bounce. Repeat the Heel Jacks in Three to the left (counts 9 through 16), cueing as: Left, Bounce, Right, Bounce, Left, Bounce, Left, Bounce. The Heel Jack in Three can be done fast by leaving out all of the even numbered counts (all of the bounces with feet together).

Heel Tilt

Begin with feet together. Touch the right heel forward while tilting the body back slightly and bending the left knee for the first count. The weight is on the left foot. Step the right foot next to the left to return to beginning

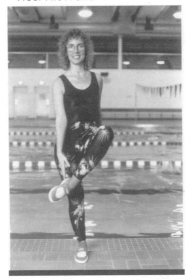

– Heel Hit Front

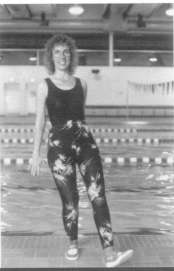

– Heel Jack

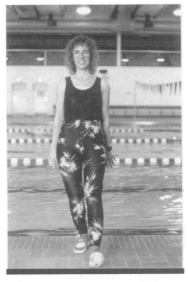

– Heel Tilt

position for the second count. Touch the left heel forward while tilting the body back slightly and bending the right knee for the third count. The weight is on the right foot. Step the left foot next to the right to return to beginning position for the fourth count. This is one set of Heel Tilts. Press both arms down and back as the heel touches forward and return to slight abduction at the sides of the body as the feet step together. To involve more abdominal work press both arms forward as in Safe Arms as the heel touches forward. The Heel Tilt works abdominals and tibialis anterior. Fast Heel Tilts are done by leaving out counts two and four, and touching the left heel out as the right heel is returning. During fast Heel Tilts punch the left arm

forward through the water while the right heel touches forward, and punch the right arms forward as the left heel touches.

Heel Turns

Begin with feet in stride position. Touch the heel of the right foot to the pool bottom in stride position with the toes of the right foot pointed to the right (external hip rotation). This is the first count of heel turns right. Touch the toes of the right foot to the pool bottom in stride position with the heel of the right foot pointed to the right (internal hip rotation). This is the second count of heel turns right. Touch the heel of the right foot to the pool bottom in stride position with the toes of the right foot pointed to the right (external hip rotation). This is

the third count of heel turns right. Bounce both feet together for the fourth count of heel turns right. This is one half set of heel turns. Touch the heel of the left foot to the pool bottom in stride position with the toes of the left foot pointed to the left (external hip rotation). This is the first count of heel turns left. Touch the toes of the left foot to the pool bottom in stride position with the heel of the left foot pointed to the left (internal hip rotation). This is the second count of heel turns left. Touch the heel of the left foot to the pool bottom in stride position with the toes of the left foot pointed to the left (external hip rotation). This is the third count of heel turns left. Bounce both feet together for the fourth count of heel turns left. This is one full set of heel turns. Flag arms with the right forearm coming up and the left forearm going down as the right heel touches and the right forearm going down and the left forearm going up as the right toe touches for heel turns right, and the left arm going up and the right arm going down as the left heel touches and the left arm going down and the right arm going up as the left toe touches for heel turns left work well with heel turns. Heel turns work the hip rotators, adductors, abductors, gastrocnemius and tibialis anterior. Heel turns can be varied

– Heel Turns (position 1)

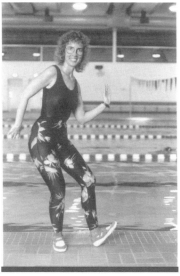

– Heel Turns (position 2)

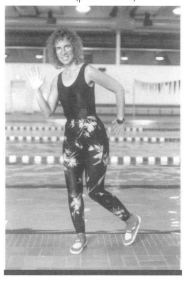

by using Heel Turn Doubles and Singles. The heel turns right would be two heel touches, two toe touches, followed by the heel turns right described above. Heel turns left would be two heel touches, two toe touches, followed by the heel turns left described above. They would be cued as "heel, heel, toe, heel, toe, heel, bounce" or "out, out, in, in, out, in, out, bounce".

Hip Flexor Stretch
See Iliopsoas Stretch

Hoedown
Begin in stride position with hips externally rotated (toes and knees pointed out). Bounce once on the right foot while the left foot pulls up behind the knee of the right leg. Bounce once on the left foot while the right foot pulls up behind the left knee. This is one set of hoedowns. The hoedown works hamstrings and quadriceps. Both arms swing laterally to the right as the left foot pulls behind the right knee, and swing to the left as the right foot moves. This move can be varied by doing two hoedowns with the left foot before changing to the right foot...this is called Hoedown Doubles. Another variation is Hoedown In Three is done by doing one set of hoedowns (left and right), two hoedowns left, one set of hoedowns (right and left) and then two hoedowns right.

Hop
Begin with feet in stride position and the body weight over the right foot and the left heel lifted back (knee flexion). Jump forward on the right leg four times. This is four hops forward and is the first four counts of this move. Reverse and hop forward four times on the left foot for the last four counts of the move. Hops can move laterally to the right or left or backwards also. Increasing the distance covered during one hop increases the intensity of the move. Hops work the gastrocnemius, quadriceps and hamstrings, but are primarily used to increase aerobic effort.

Hopscotch
Begin by bouncing once in stride position. This is the first count. For the second count bounce once on the right foot while the left heel pulls up behind the right thigh. Bounce once in stride position with both feet down for the third count. For the fourth count bounce on the left foot while the right heel pulls up behind the left thigh. This is one set of Hopscotch. This move works the quadriceps and hamstrings. Arms begin extended laterally. The right arm presses down through the water toward the left heel as the heel pulls up behind the right thigh. Arms return to the beginning position for the third count. For the fourth count, the left arm presses down through the water toward the right heel.

–Hoedown

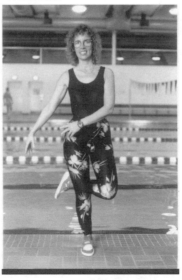

– Hopscotch

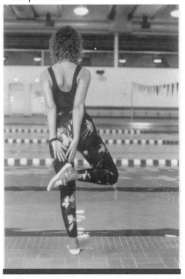

Iliopsoas (Hip Flexor) Stretch
Stand facing pool edge, holding the pool edge with the left hand for support. Reach behind the body with the right hand and grasp the right lower leg near the ankle. Push the right hip forward by contracting the right gluteals. The knee will be pointed back about one inch. By pointing the toes up, this is also an Anterior Tibialis stretch. Another variation to stretch the iliopsoas is to stand in a gastrocnemius stretch position and move into a pelvic tilt. The heel of the back foot will lift off the pool bottom as the knee pushes forward during the pelvic tilt.

Jazzkick
Begin in stride position. With hip extended, flex (bend) the right knee pulling the heel back toward the buttocks. This is the first count. Extend (straighten) the right knee and slightly flex (bend) the hip. This is the second count. Repeat with the left leg. This move works the quadriceps and hamstrings. It can be varied by kicking to the diagonal (with hips externally rotated) or kicking several times with one leg before switching to the other. Jog arms work with the Jazzkick. Using both arms in a flexed arm stroke and backstroke move also works well.

Jazzkick Diagonals
Begin with jazzkicks forward, alternating right and left feet. Externally rotate the hips while continuing the jazzkicks. The jazzkicks should now be kicking to the right diagonal with the right foot and kicking to the left diagonal with the left foot.

Jig
Begin with weight on left foot

– Jazzkick (position 1)

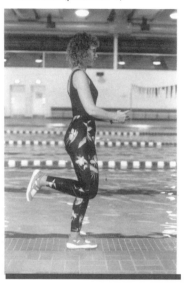

– Iliopsoas (Hip Flexor) Stretch (position 1)

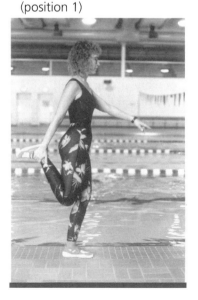

– Iliopsoas (Hip Flexor) Stretch (position 2)

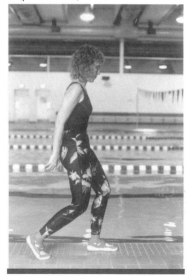

– Jazzkick (position 1)

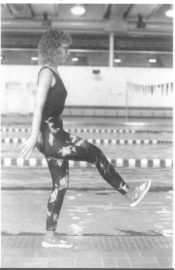

and right heel extended to the right and touching the pool bottom. The toes on the right foot are pointed to the right. The right heel pulls up in front of the left knee for the first count. Return to beginning position for the second count. The right heel pulls up behind the left knee for the third count. Move to stride position (feet about shoulder width apart) for the fourth count. Repeat with the left leg or repeat three more times with the right leg before doing the move four times with the left leg. This move works the quadriceps and hamstrings. Adduct the left arm down through the water in front and behind the body toward the right heel as it comes up in front and behind the left knee. The right arm adducts down through the water behind and then in front of the body (opposite the left arm).

Jog Arms

Jog arms work biceps and triceps. Elbows are in at the waist and forearms down at sides (arm and elbow extension). The right forearm comes up and forward (elbow flexion) as a step is taken on the left foot. The right arm returns to beginning position (elbow extension) while the left arm comes up and forward (elbow flexion) as a step is taken on the right foot.

Jog Doubles

Begin with feet in stride position. Step forward on the right foot while lifting the left off the pool bottom for the first count. Bounce once on the right foot while keeping the left foot off the pool bottom for the second count. Step forward on the left foot while lifting the right foot off the pool bottom for the third count. Bounce once on the left foot while keeping the right foot off the pool bottom for the fourth count. This is one set of

– Jig (position 1)

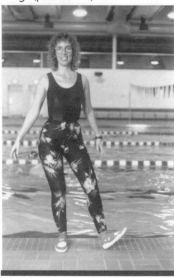

– Jig (position 3)

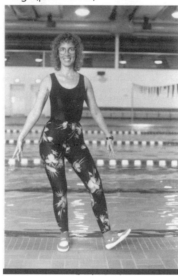

– Jig (position 2)

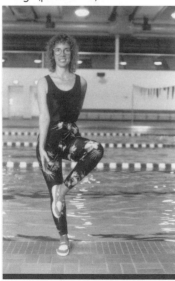

– Jig (position 4)

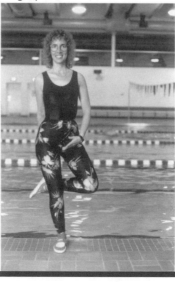

jog doubles. Jog doubles can be done in place or moved forward and back. They work the gastrocnemius.

Jog Tilt

Lean the entire body slightly forward keeping the body straight (eliminate any spinal flexion that causes a bend at the waist) and jog forward. Lean the entire body slightly back, keeping the body straight and jog backwards. The tilt in the body is extremely small. This move works ilipsoas, gluteals and abdominals. Jog arms or small stroke and backstroke arms work well with the Jog Tilt.

Jump Bounce

Jump bounces move forward and back and can be done singly with one jump bounce moving forward and one jump bounce moving back or in series with 4 or 8 jump bounces moving forward followed by 4 or 8 jump bounces moving back. Begin in a closed stride position. Jump forward as far as possible with a big jump for the first count. Bounce in place with a small bounce for the second count. This is one jump bounce moving forward. Jump backwards covering as much distance as possible with a big jump for the first count of a jump bounce back. Bounce in place with a small bounce for the second count of jump bounce back. Safe arms pushing back as the jump bounce forward is accomplished and pushing forward as the jump bounce back is done work well with this move. If done slowly, participants can increase the intensity by tucking the knees to the chest during the big jump as the first count of jump bounce forward and jump bounce back. The jump bounce works iliopsoas, gluteals and gastrocnemius, but is usually used for increasing aerobic training.

Jumping Jacks

Begin with feet in stride position. Jump both feet out to the sides into a wide stride position. Jump both feet together. This is one Jumping Jack. Arms can press down behind, press down in front, press down with elbows flexed, or arms can be out of the water pushing up or flying out and up. Jumping Jacks can be done "in 3" by jumping out, in, out, out, and then in, out, in, in. Jumping Jacks work the adductors and abductors. Jumping Jacks can be done moving forward and back or right and left to vary the intensity.

Jumping Jack Crossing

Begin with feet in stride position. Jump both feet out to the sides into a wide stride position. Jump both feet together with the right foot crossed over (in front and to the left of) the left foot. Jump both feet out to the sides into a wide stride position. Jump both feet together with the

– Jog Tilt (position 1)

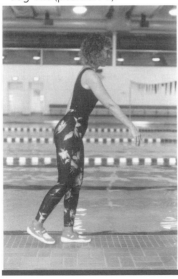

– Jog Tilt   (position 2)

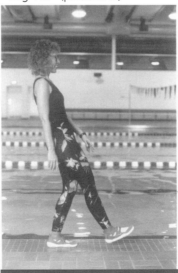

left foot crossed over (in front and to the right of) the right foot. This is one set of Jumping Jacks Crossing. Arms press down with one arm in front of the body and one behind. The left arm should press in front of the body when the right foot is crossed over the left, and the right arm should press in front of the body when the left foot is crossed over the right. This move works adductors, abductors, deltoids and latissimus dorsi.

Jumping Jack Doubles
Begin with feet in stride position. Jump both feet apart and out to the sides into a wide stride position for the first count. Bounce once with both feet in the wide stride position for the second count. Jump both feet

together for the third count. Bounce once with both feet together for the fourth count. This is one set of Jumping Jack Doubles. This move works adductors and abductors. See Jumping Jacks for arm variations. The Jumping Jack Doubles can varied by moving them forward and back or right and left, or by pulling both knees up (in the position they're in) between each count.

Jumping Jack Jump
Also called Split Jumps. Begin with feet together. Jump high while abducting legs and then adducting legs (legs move apart and out to sides and then come back together) before landing again with feet in beginning position. This is one jump. Jump-

ing Jack Jumps work adductors and abductors and should be used only with well conditioned students. Any arms that help to maintain proper body alignment can be used. Arms that follow the legs out and in (a reverse press down) work well.

Karate Punch
Begin with elbows in toward waist, elbows flexed at about a 90 degree angle and forearms forward. Make fists. Punch right arm across to the left until arm is extended. While pulling the right elbow back to beginning position, punch the left arm forward until arm is extended. Continue punching the right arm to the left to a count of "one" and following that with a forward punch of the left arm

– Jumping Jack Crossing (position 1)

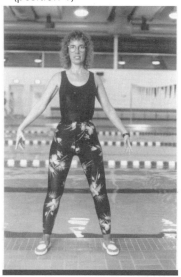

– Jumping Jack Crossing (position 2)

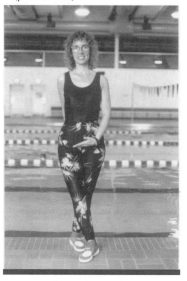

– Jumping Jack Jump

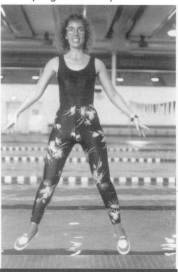

to a count of "two". Reverse by punching the left arm across to the right and punching the right arm forward. This move works the pectorals, deltoids, biceps, triceps, trapezius and rhomboids. Feet, knees and hips should pivot to the left when the right arm is punching to the left, and, conversely, they should pivot to the right when the left arm is punching to the right. When punching forward, feet should be in the forward stride position. Participants can bounce from one position to the next or simply pivot easily on the balls of the feet.

Kick

Begin with feet in stride position and lift the right leg (hip flexion) forward. Return that leg to beginning position (hip extension) and lift the left leg forward. Kicks can be done fast, lifting one leg while lowering the other, or they can be done slow by bouncing both feet together before doing the next kick. Maintain proper body alignment during kicks, keeping shoulders slightly back and the torso tall. Students will want to lean forward to kick higher. This should be discouraged. This move works the iliopsoas and gluteals.

Kick Corner

Also called Kick Diagonal. Begin with feet in stride position with hips slightly externally rotated. Lift the right leg to the right diagonal, return it to beginning position, and lift the left leg to the left diagonal. As with forward kicks, kicks to the corner can be done slow or fast. The same precautions apply. Corner kicks work the iliopsoas and gluteals.

Kick Point and Flex

Kick forward 4 or 8 times with the toe pointed forward (plantar flexed) and then kick forward the same amount of times with the toe pointed up toward the body (dorsi flexed). This move works the gastrocnemius, anterior tibialis, iliopsoas and gluteals. The kicks can be fast or slow as described in Kick, and can be forward or diagonal kicks.

Kickswing

Begin with feet in stride position. Kick the right foot forward

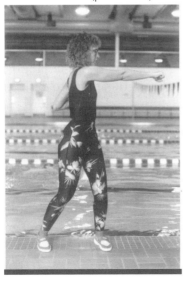
– Karate Punch (position 1)

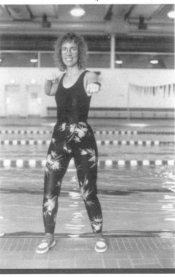
– Karate Punch   (position 2)

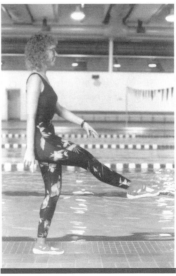
– Kick Point and Flex

(hip flexion) as high as possible for the first count. Swing the right leg back into slight hip hyperextension (just past returning to beginning position) while bouncing once on the left leg for the second count. This is one Kickswing Right. Repeat counts one and two 3 more times before switching to Kickswing Left for 4 times. The Kickswing works the iliopsoas and gluteals. To protect the low back, abdominals should be contracted and the body should be in a pelvic tilt during the "swing" portion of the move. Swing the right arm back and the left arm forward as the right leg kicks forward. Swing the right arm forward and the left arm back as the left leg kicks back. Reverse for the Kickswing Left.

– Kick and Flex

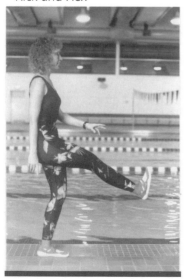

Kneelift

Begin with feet in stride position. Lift the right leg (hip flexion) to approximately a 90 degree angle while bending the right knee (knee flexion) to about a 90 degree angle. Repeat with the left leg. Kneelifts can be done fast, lifting one leg while lowering the other (which is very much like a jog with high-lifting knees), or they can be done slow by bouncing both feet together before doing the next kneelift. Kneelifts can be alternated, right and then left, or repeated 2,4 or 8 times on the right leg before changing to the left. They can be moved to the right and left to increase the intensity. Kneelifts work the iliopsoas and gluteals.

– Kneelift Cross

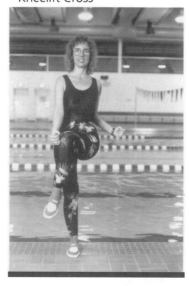

Kneelift Cross

Begin with feet in stride position with the right hip slightly internally rotated (toes and knees pointed inward). Pull the right knee up toward the left shoulder without allowing the shoulders to move forward. Return the right leg to beginning position and repeat 1,3 or 7 more times. Repeat with the left leg. Crossing knee-lifts work the iliopsoas, gluteals, abductors and adductors. Touch the left wrist to the inside (internal aspect) of the right knee and reverse. Trying to touch the left elbow to the right knee can result in simultaneous flexion and rotation of the spine which is contraindicated. Touching the wrist to the elbow allows the spine to stay erect (extended) while the spinal rotation occurs.

Kneelift Out

Begin in stride position with both hips externally rotated (knees and toes pointed out). Pull the right knee up to the right diagonal while keeping the torso tall (not tilting to the left). Return the right leg and repeat with the left. Kneelifts out (also called Open Kneelifts) can be done fast or slow, or in groups of 2, 4 or 8 as described in KNEELIFTS. This move works iliopsoas and gluteals. Both arms push down in front or press down behind.

Kneeswing Crossing

Begin with the right knee flexed to a 90 degree angle (knee bent) and hip flexed to a 90 degree angle so the knee is pointed forward and lower leg is straight down. Weight is on left foot. Cross knee to the left (internally rotate the hip) while maintaining hip and knee flexion. This is the first count. Swing the knee out to the right side (externally rotate the hip) while maintaining hip and knee flexion. This is the second count. Both arms push laterally to the right as the knee crosses to the left, and push to the left as the knee swings out to the right. Crossing kneeswings can be done in groups of 2, 4 or 8 with the right leg before repeating with the left leg. Kneeswing crossing works hip abductors and adductors.

Kneeswing Combo

This is a combination of the Kneeswing Up and Back and the Crossing Kneeswing. Do one set of Kneeswing Up and Back (swing right knee up, back, up and then set right foot down; swing left knee up, back, up and then set left foot down). Follow that with one set of Crossing Kneeswing (right knee crosses, opens, crosses and then set right foot down; left knee crosses, opens, crosses and then set left foot down). This is one set of Kneeswing Combo. Kneeswings can be also be combined by doing Kneeswing Up and Back 4 times with the right leg, then 4 times with the left leg, Crossing Kneeswing 4 times with the right leg, and then 4 times with the left leg. They can also be combined doing 2 Kneeswings Up and Back and 2 Crossing Kneeswings on the right leg, and then repeating on the left leg.

Kneeswing Diagonal

This is a Kneeswing Up and Back with the hip slightly rotated externally so that the knee is pointed to the diagonal.

Kneeswing Up and Back

Begin with the right knee flexed to an 90 degree angle (knee bent) and hip extended so the knee is pointed straight down. Weight is on the left foot. Swing right knee forward keeping knee flexed at a 90 degree angle. This is the first count. Swing right knee back (while maintaining the knee flexion) to a slight hip hyperextension. This is the second count. Left arm swings forward as right knee swings for-

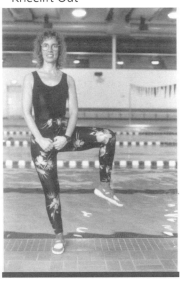

– Kneelift Out

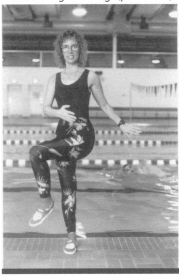

– Kneeswing Crossing (position 1)

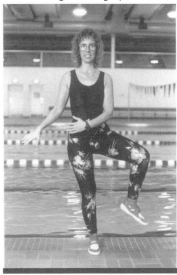

– Kneeswing Crossing (position 2)

ward, and back as the right knee swings back. Kneeswing right can be repeated 1,3 or 7 times more before changing to

– Kneeswing Up and Back (position 1)

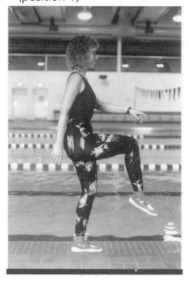

kneeswings left. This move works the iliopsoas and gluteals. It can be moved forward and back to increase the intensity.

Lateral Push
Right arm begins extended laterally to the right with palm down (pronated). Left arm begins adducted across the body so that the left hand is about parallel with the right elbow. Palm of the left hand is facing down (pronated) also. Both arms are near the top of the water surface. To accomplish the lateral push, press both arms down and to the left until they are near the top of the water surface on the left side. Reverse to move in the opposite direction. This is an excellent move to use when moving laterally through the water. Arms push to the left

when the body is moving right. The lateral push works deltoids, latissimus dorsi, trapezius and pectorals.

Leap Forward
Begin with the arms forward just below the water surface with palms out and knuckles almost touching. Kick the right foot forward and jump forward onto it as arms push out and back. Bring the left foot next to the right while bringing the arms forward again. Repeat the leap with the right foot three more times and then repeat it four times with the left foot leading. Jog or bounce backward to return to beginning position. If the pool does not allow enough space to leap four forward with the right foot and four forward with the left foot, participants

– Kneeswing Up and Back (position 2)

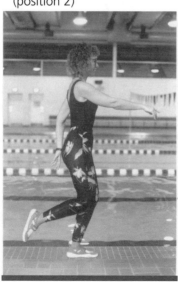

– Lateral Push

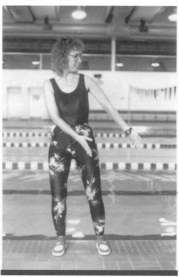

– Leap Forward (position 1)

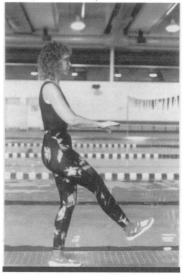

can leap two forward with the right foot and two forward with the left foot or leap forward four times with the right foot leading, then turn a half-turn left and return with the left foot leading. This move works the iliopsoas, pectorals, trapezius and gluteals.

Leap Side

Begin with weight on left foot, arms both extended laterally (out to the side) to the right, and right leg slightly lifted out to the side (abducted). Jump the right leg to the right as far as possible while still facing forward and while both arms push down and to the left. This is the first count. Bring the left foot (adduct) next to right and bounce both feet together. This is the second count. During the second count the arms return to beginning position. Repeat counts one and two three more times while moving to the right. To reverse the leap, begin with the left foot jumping out to the left and move left. While moving to the left both arms extend laterally to the left and push down and to the right during the jump to the left during the first count. Leap Side works adductors and abductors. The toes of both feet should continually face forward, not the sides, to ensure adductor and abductor work. Leading the step with the heel will help to ensure proper forward alignment of the hips. The Leap Side can be modified to work obliques by tightening the hips with the legs in the leap position, concentrating on moving from the waist and keeping the upper torso stable.

Lift Hips

Begin with back to pool edge, elbows up on pool edge, hips flexed at 90 degrees so that the knees are pointing forward, and knees flexed at 90 degrees so that the feet are hanging down. The back must be flat to the pool wall. Slowly contract abdominal muscles so that knees move forward an inch or two. This will move the very low back and hips away from the pool edge. Return the back to beginning position without allowing the middle of the back to move away from the pool wall. This move works abdominals. If done incorrectly with the knees moving up and down rather than forward and back the move will work the iliopsoas muscles. If the hip joint is moving (flexing and extending) the move is in-

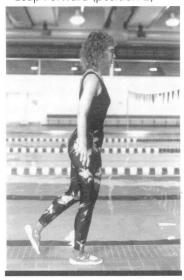

– Leap Forward (position 2)

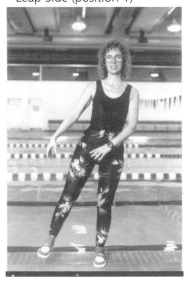

– Leap Side (position 1)

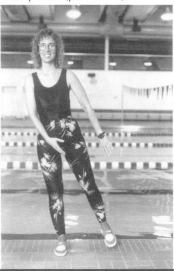

– Leap Side (position 2)

– Lift Hips

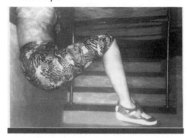

correct. If the spine is moving the move is correct and the abdominals will be working. This move can be modified by changing the degree of flexion in the knees and hips.

Mule Kicks

Mule kicks can be done "fast" (without a bounce between each kick) or "slow" (with a bounce between each kick). Mule kicks are simple knee flexion (trying to kick the heel up to the buttocks) while keeping the knee pointed straight down (hip flexors extended). Mule kicks can be done alternating right and then left, or four to eight can be done with the right leg before changing to the left. Mule kicks work quadriceps and hamstrings. Optional arms include Elbow Press and Scissor arms. Two other arm variations: 1. Beginning with elbows flexed at about a 90 degree angle and elbows pulled in to waist with forearms forward, lift both elbows laterally as the heel kicks behind, and lower as the foot returns. These arms can also be done with the arms beginning straight down at the sides of the body. 2. Beginning with arms down in front of body with palms on thighs, make fists and lift both arms forward as the heel kicks behind, and lower as the foot returns.

Neck Stretch

Tilt the head to the right side, moving the right ear to the right shoulder. Reverse for neck stretch left.

Oblique Stretch

Stand with feet shoulder width apart. Toes should be pointed slightly out, and knees slightly bent. Put left hand on left hip and extend right arm up and over the head without moving the toes or knees. This should stretch the obliques. If further stretch is required, slowly bend sideways toward the hand on the hip.

Over and Present

Begin with arms extended laterally (out to the sides) up to just

– Mule Kick

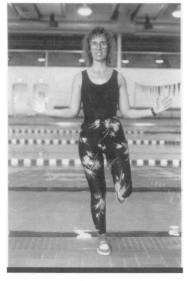

– Neck Stretch

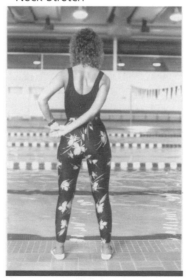

– Oblique Stretch

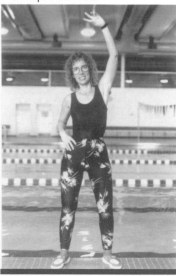

beneath the water surface with palms forward. With elbow extended so arm is straight, bring right hand toward left until almost touching. Turn palm out (externally rotated) and push extended right arm back to beginning position. This can be repeated with the right arm several times before switching to the left or it can be done alternating right and left. This works pectorals, anterior serratus, trapezius, rhomboids and lattisimus dorsi. To maintain integrity of the knee joint pivot each foot to follow the knee. To use this move to work the obliques, stand with feet shoulder width apart and move only from the waist up. Knees should be slightly flexed and both knees and toes should be pointed slightly out.

Paddlekick

This move is done in a floating position with back to pool edge with elbows on pool edge, buoyant hand bars in hands or under each arm. With hips flexed (bent) at a 90 degree angle and knees flexed at a 90 degree angle so feet hang down, alternately extend each knee while keeping both knees on the same plane. This move works quadriceps and hamstrings.

Pectoral Stretch

With fingers interlaced behind the head and elbows pointed out to the sides, squeeze shoulder blades together. See also Bicep, Anterior Deltoid and Pectoral Stretch.

Pelvic Tilt

Begin by standing in a comfortable upright position. Create a pelvic tilt using one or more of these imagery techniques: pull the naval back to the spine, press the stomach down toward the pool bottom, tuck the buttocks under, or take the arch out of the low back. This is one pelvic tilt. The pelvic tilt can be used during many exercise moves to protect the low back from strain. A series of 8 to 24 standing pelvic tilts can be used during the toning portion of the workout. The pelvic tilt works the abdominal muscles.

Press Down Behind

Begin with arms laterally extended (lifted to the sides) just

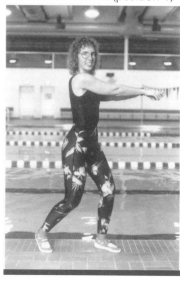

– Over and Present (position 1)

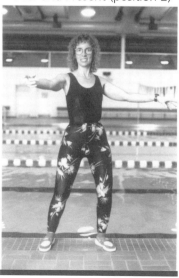

– Over and Present (position 2)

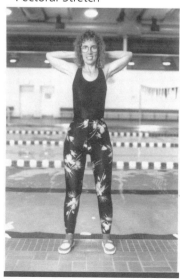

– Pectoral Stretch

beneath the water surface with palms down (pronated). Push both arms down through the water until they almost meet behind the body. This portion of the move focuses on latissimus dorsi and trapezius. To reverse the Press Down simply keep palms down and lift the arms with force through the water to beginning position. This portion of the move focuses on deltoids. When used for toning the arms should stop (pause momentarily) between the Press Down and the reverse portion of the move.

Press Down Front
Begin with arms extended laterally (lifted out to the sides) just beneath the water surface with palms down (pronated). Push

both arms down through the water until they almost meet in front of the body. This portion of the move focuses on pectorals and serratus anterior. To reverse the Press Down simply keep palms down and lift the arms with force through the water to beginning position. This portion of the move focuses on deltoids. When used for toning the arms should stop (pause momentarily) between each portion of the move.

Press Down Singles
Begin with arms extended laterally (lifted out to the sides) just beneath the water surface with palms down (pronated). Press the right arm down as described in Press Down Front while pressing the left arm down as

described in Press Down Behind. Reverse the move also as described. To continue the move press the left arm down in front and the right arm down behind, and lift them both to beginning position. This is one set of Press Down Singles. Deltoids, pectorals, serratus anterior, latissimus dorsi and trapezius are all involved in this move.

Press Down with Elbows Flexed
Begin with elbows extended laterally (lifted out to the sides) and forearms forward (90 to 120 degree elbow flexion) with palms down. The arms should begin just below the water surface. Push both arms down through the water until forearms almost meet in front of the body. This portion of the move works the

– Pelvic Tilt
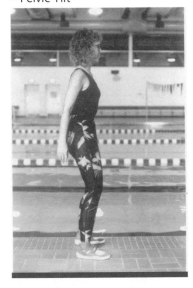

– Press Down Behind
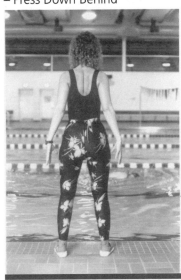

– Press Down with Elbows Flexed
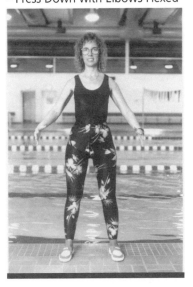

pectorals and serratus anterior. To reverse, lift the arms with force back to beginning position. The reverse portion of the move works deltoids and trapezius.

Quadricep Stretch
Stand facing pool edge. Hold the pool edge with the left hand for support. Reach behind the body with right hand and grasp the right lower leg near the ankle. Pull the right lower leg and heel gently toward the right buttocks. Knee should point directly to the pool bottom and toe should also be pointed straight down. Reverse for left quadricep stretch.

Reach Pull-In
Begin with both arms extended laterally out to the side just beneath the water surface to the left at shoulder level. Feet, knees, hips and shoulders are pivoted to the left to allow the palms to begin in a parallel position. This is the "reach" position of this move. While pivoting feet, knees and hips forward, pull both elbows back until shoulder blades are squeezed together. This is the "pull in" portion of the move. Continue to the left before switching to the right or alternate by doing one left and then one right. Reach Pull-In involves the pectorals, deltoids, trapezius and rhomboids. It can be done bouncing into the pivot and back to the forward position or simply by pivoting lightly with no bounce.

Reverse Crossing Jog
Reverse crossing jog moves laterally to the right with four to eight steps before moving laterally to the left with four or eight steps. Begin with feet in stride position. Step the right foot laterally to the right. Shift the weight to the right foot while lifting the left leg slightly up off the pool bottom. This is the first count of reverse crossing jog right. Step the left foot behind the right foot, shifting the weight to the left foot while lifting the right foot up slightly for the second count. Repeat counts one and two three to seven times while moving to the right. Step the left foot laterally to the left. Shift the weight to the left foot while the right foot comes up

– Quadricep Stretch

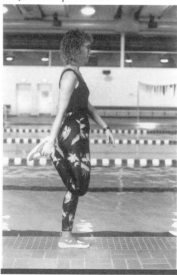

– Reach Pull-In (position 1)

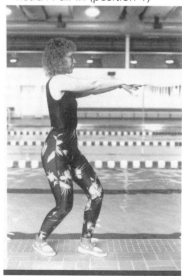

– Reach Pull-In (position 2)

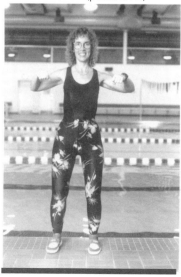

slightly off the pool bottom. This is the first count of reverse crossing jog left. Step the right foot behind the left foot, shifting the weight to the right foot and slightly lifting the left foot up. This is the second count of reverse crossing jog left. Repeat three to seven times more while moving to the left. Arms can stay on hips or can push laterally to the right when moving left and push laterally to the left when moving right. Keep the torso facing forward to achieve the excellent oblique, adductor and abductor work the crossing jog provides. The crossing jog can also be done with the leading foot crossing behind instead of in front as described above. While moving left, the right foot would step behind the left foot for the first count of each two count segment. While moving right, the left foot would behind the right foot during the first count of each two count segment. This is called crossing jog behind and also works the adductors and abductors. The crossing jog in front and behind can be combined to create a grapevine move. A two count segment of crossing jog in front would be followed by a two count segment of crossing jog behind moving left and repeated twice before reversing to move to the right. This can be called a crossing jog combo or a grapevine. The cues would be "cross, step, back, step, cross, step, back, step".

Rhomboid Stretch
Place palms on center of the upper back and press elbows together.

Rock in Three
Begin with the weight on the left foot and the right foot abducted (slightly lifted out to the right side). This is the first count. For the second count, step the right foot down as the left foot lifts out to the left side. Step the left foot down as the right foot lifts out to the right side (beginning position) for the third count. For the fourth count pivot slightly to the right on the left foot and kick the right leg to the right. Step the right foot down as the left foot lifts out the left side for the fifth count. Step the left foot down as the right foot

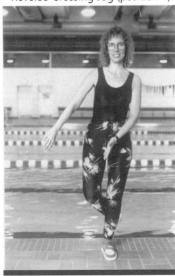

– Reverse Crossing Jog (position 1)

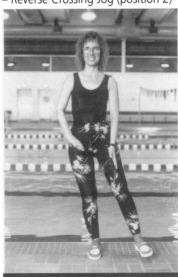

– Reverse Crossing Jog (position 2)

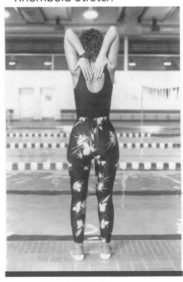

– Rhomboid Stretch

lifts out to the right side (beginning position) for the sixth count. Step the right foot down as the left foot lifts out to the left side for the seventh count. For the eighth count pivot slightly to the left on the right foot and kick the left leg to the left. This is one set of Rock in Three. This move works adductors, abductors, iliopsoas and gluteals.

Rock Side to Side

Begin with the weight on the left foot and the right foot abducted (slightly lifted out to the right side). Step the right foot down as the left foot lifts out to the left side. This is one set of Rock Side to Side. Arms can Press Down alternately or can Lateral Push to the left as the right leg rocks out and push to the right as the left leg rocks out. The Rock Side to Side works adductors and abductors. Lead the rocking with the heel to assist in keeping the toes of both feet pointing forward continually and the hips in forward alignment. The Rock Side to Side can be modified to work obliques by tightening the hip joints with legs in a rocking position, concentrating on moving from the waist and keeping the upper body stable.

Rockinghorse

Begin with the weight on the left foot and the right foot lifted (hip flexion) slightly in front of it's standing position. Step the right foot forward and lean the body forward over the right foot while keeping the body straight. Avoid any spinal flexion that might cause the body to bend at the waist. The left foot will come up off the pool bottom and kick slightly back as the weight is shifted to the right foot. This is the first count of Rockinghorse. Step the left foot back to beginning position and lean the body slightly back over the left foot while keeping the body straight. Avoid any spinal hyperextension that might cause the body to bend backwards at the waist. The right foot will come up off the pool bottom and kick slightly forward as the weight is shifted to the left foot. This is the second count of Rockinghorse. Repeat counts one and two 3 more times and then switch to Rockinghorse Left with the left foot rocking forward and the right foot rock-

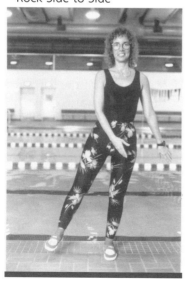

– Rock Side to Side

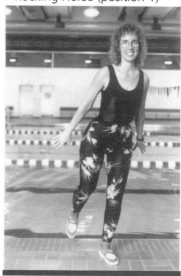

– Rocking Horse (position 1)

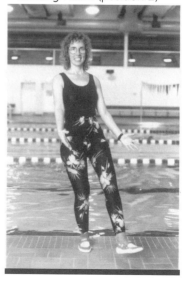

– Rocking Horse (position 2)

ing back. The Rockinghorse works iliopsoas, gluteals and abdominals. Safe Arms pushing back as the body leans (rocks) forward and pushing forward as the body rocks back work well with this move. This move can be varied by doing it to the right and left diagonals rather than forward. This is called Rockinghorse Diagonals. Lift the right leg toward the right diagonal and turn the body in that direction before stepping on the right foot for the first count. Lift the left leg toward the left diagonal and turn the body in that direction before stepping on the left foot for the second count.

Rockinghorse Doubles

Rock forward on the right foot as described in Rockinghorse for the first count. Bounce once on the right foot (keeping it in first count position) for the second count. Rock back on the left foot as described in Rockinghorse for the third count. Bounce once on the left foot (keeping it in the third count position) for the fourth count. This is one set of Rockinghorse Doubles Right. Repeat counts one through four 3 more times before switching to Rockinghorse Doubles Left with the left foot rocking forward, bouncing, and then the right foot rocking back and bouncing. The Rockinghorse Doubles work ilipsoas, gluteals and abdominals. Safe Arms

work well with this move. These can also be varied by rocking to the diagonals.

Rockinghorse in Three

Rock forward on the right foot as described in Rockinghorse for the first count. Rock back on the left foot as described in Rockinghorse for the second count. Rock forward on the right foot to return to first count position. Kick the left foot forward as the body returns to up-right position for the fourth count. (This much of the move is called Rockinghorse in Three Right.) Rock forward on the left foot for the fifth count, back on the right for the sixth count, and forward on the left for the seventh count. Kick the right foot forward as the body returns to upright position for the eighth count. (This portion of the move is called Rockinghorse in Three Left.) The combination of everything done so far is one set of Rockinghorse in Three. This move works the iliopsoas, gluteals and abdominals. Safe Arms work well with this move. This move can be combined with Rockinghorse Doubles for a move called Rockinghorse Three and Doubles. Do a Rockinghorse in Three Right, a Rockinghorse Doubles Left, a Rockinghorse in Three Left, and a Rockinghorse Doubles Right. This is one set of Rockinghorse Three and Doubles. Students

can learn well with these cues on the beats: "up, back, up, kick, up, up, back, back" (these words would be repeated twice for one full set of Rockinghorse Three and Doubles) OR "right, left, right, kick, left, left, right, right; left, right, left, kick, right, right, left, left." These can also be varied by using Rockinghorse Diagonals.

Rockinghorse Seven and Up

Rock forward on the right foot as described in Rockinghorse for the first count. Rock back on the left foot as described in Rockinghorse for the second count. Rock forward on the right foot for the third count, back on the left foot for the fourth count, forward on the right foot for the fifth count, back on the left foot for the sixth count and forward on the right foot for the seventh count. Kick the left foot forward on the eighth count. This portion of the move is called Rockinghorse Seven and Up Right. Rock forward on the left foot, back on the right, forward on the left, back on the right, forward on the left, back on the right, forward on the left, and kick the right foot forward for Rockinghorse Seven and Up Left. This entire move is one set of Rockinghorse Seven and Up. This move works the iliopsoas, gluteals and abdominals. Safe Arms work well with this move. The

Rockinghorse Seven and Up can be combined with Rockinghorse Doubles for variety. The combination is called Rockinghorse Seven and Doubles. Do one set of Rockinghorse Seven and Up Right for the first eight counts, two sets of Rockinghorse Doubles Left for the second eight counts, one set of Rockinghorse Seven and Up Left for the third eight counts, and two sets of Rockinghorse Doubles Right for the fourth eight counts. This is one set of Rockinghorse Seven and Doubles. These can also be varied by using Rockinghorse Diagonals.

Russian Kicks

With hips and knees flexed (bent) as much as possible (almost in a sitting position in the pool) alternately extend each knee without changing the degree of hip flexion. Students must be in shallower water to accomplish this move successfully. Russian Kicks work quadriceps, hamstrings and gluteals. Arms can be in a folded position in front of chest like the Russian dancers or they can punch alternately in opposition to the kicks.

Safe Arms

Begin with arms extended laterally out to the sides with palms forward. Arms are just beneath the water surface. With elbows extended so arms are straight,

bring hands together in front of body. Turn palms back and, with straight arms, bring hands together (or as close as possible) behind body. This move works pectorals, anterior serratus, trapezius, rhomboids and lattisimus dorsi. Rockinghorses, and forward and back Lunges work well with Safe Arms.

Scissor Arms

Begin with arms extended laterally with palms down. With elbows extended so arms are straight, push arms straight down in front of body until palms meet. With shoulders back and palms still down, pull arms up with force to beginning position. This move can be varied by crossing the hands in the lowered position in front of the

body. This increases the range of motion involved in the movement. The serratus anterior, pectorals, lattisimus dorsi, deltoids and trapezius are all involved in this move. These arms can be used in Jumping Jacks and most lateral movements such as Side Step and Side Kick.

Scissors

Bounce into a cross country ski position with the right foot at least twelve inches in front of the left. Bounce into the reverse position with the left foot in front of the right. When the right foot is forward the left arm should swing or punch forward and reverse. This move can be varied by having the toes of the forward foot pointed up (dorsiflexed) while tilting the body slightly back. It can also

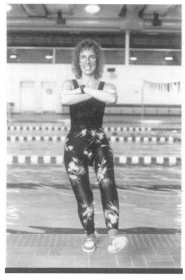

– Russian Kick

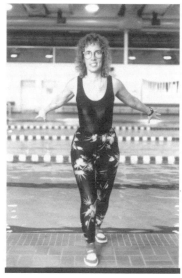

– Safe Arms

95

be varied by pointing the toes of the back foot down while tilting the body slightly forward. Scissors can be done moving forward, back or in a circle to increase the intensity. Scissors work the iliopsoas and gluteals. Tilting back with the front foot toes dorsiflexed focuses work on the iliopsoas and also involves the tibialis anterior and abdominals. Tilting forward with the back foot toes down focuses work on the gluteals and involves the gastrocnemius.

Scissors Jump
Also called Vertical Jumps. Jump into a cross country ski position with the right foot in front of the left. While still suspended in the water bring both feet together and land with feet next to each other. Jump into a cross country ski position with the left foot in front of the right. While still suspended in the water bring both feet together and land with feet next to each other. Scissor jumps work the iliopsoas, gluteals and gastrocnemius. Left arm should swing forward as the right leg goes forward and reverse. Scissor Jumps should be used in high intensity classes for well conditioned students only.

Scissors Turn
Bounce into a cross country ski position with the right foot about 12 inches in front of the left. For the second count, pivot (or bounce) 1/2 turn left keeping the feet in the same place but changing their position so that the body is facing the back of the pool. Bounce twice with feet together for counts three and four. Repeat counts one through four to face front. The Scissors Turn works iliopsoas, gluteals, gastrocnemius and obliques. The Scissor Turn can be used with quarter turns rather than half turns. Bounce into the cross country ski position as stated above. For the second count, pivot or bounce a quarter turn to the left. Bounce twice with feet together for counts three and four. To face each wall with this move, repeat counts one through four 4 times.

Scissors with Bounce
Bounce into a cross country ski position with the right foot about 12 inches in front of the left. Bounce both feet together next to each other. Bounce into a cross country ski position with

– Scissor Arms

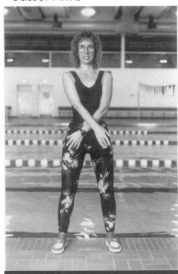

– Scissors

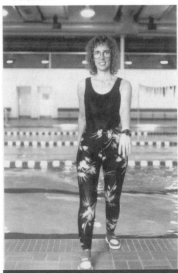

– Scissors Jump

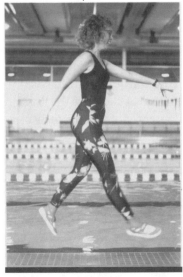

the left foot about 12 inches in front of the right. Bounce both feet together next to each other. Arms and variations written for Scissors also apply to Scissor with Bounce. This move works the iliopsoas and gluteals. The Scissors with Bounce can be varied by twisting the body so the toes of the right foot point to the right diagonal when the right foot is forward, and the toes of the left foot point to the left diagonal when the left foot is forward.

Shoulder Shrugs
Standing in stride position (with feet shoulder width apart) with arms relaxed at sides, squeeze shoulders together in front of body. Then squeeze shoulders together behind the body. Shoulder Shrugs work pectorals, deltoids, trapezius and rhomboids. They can be done with moves like Jumping Jacks or alone for joint lubrication during the warm up.

Side Circle
Begin standing at pool edge, holding pool edge to stabilize body. Weight is on the left foot with right leg straight down and right foot next to the left foot. Extend the right leg back (hip hyperextension) and circle the leg out to the side, around to the front and back to beginning position. Repeat 7 more times and reverse. During the "reverse" the right leg will move forward (hip

flexion), circle out to the side and around to the back before returning to beginning position. Repeat the Side Circles back and forward with the left leg. The Side Circles work adductors, abductors, iliopsoas and gluteals. As the leg circles the body should remain in good alignment. If the upper body is moving around, the leg circles should be smaller. This is a toning move and not used during the aerobic portion of the workout.

Side Kick
Begin in stride position. Abduct (lift out to the side) the right leg while bouncing once on the left leg for the first count. Return the right leg to beginning position (adduct) and bounce on both feet for the second count. Abduct the left leg while bouncing once on the right leg for the third count. Return the left leg to beginning position and bounce on both feet for the fourth count. This is one set of Side Kicks. The Side Kick works adductors and abductors. Properly position the leg with the toes pointing forward and the heel pointing slightly out to the right before kicking out to the right. The Side Kick can be varied by doing 2, 4 or 8 with the right leg before switching to the left leg. Press Down Behind and Press Down Front arms both work well with the Side Kick.

Side Kick Forward and Back
Begin in stride position. Abduct (lift out to the side) the right leg and bounce once on the left leg for the first count. Adduct (return toward the other leg) the right leg to just in front of the left ankle while bouncing once on the left leg for the second count. Abduct the right leg while bouncing once on the left leg for the third count. Adduct the right leg to just behind the left ankle while bouncing once on the left leg for the fourth count. This is one Side Kick Forward and Back. If used during the toning portion of the workout it should be repeated 4 or 8 times before switching to the left leg. If used during the aerobics portion it should be done only once on the right leg before switching to the left leg.

– Sidekick Forward

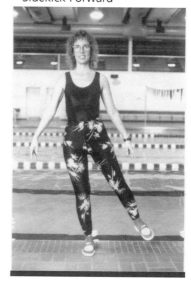

97

The Side Kick Forward and Back works adductors and abductors. If used during the aerobics portion, Press Down the left arm in front of the body (and the right arm behind) when the right leg is adducted in front of the left ankle and Press Down the right arm in front of the body (and the left arm behind) when the left leg is adducted behind the right ankle. Side Kick Forward and Back works adductors and abductors.

Side Lift
The side lift is a toning move which is a side kick done without the bounce.

Side Lift Flex
This is a Side Kick with the knee slightly flexed. It is used during the toning portion of the workout and students should be holding pool edge for stability. With the knee pointing straight down (hip extension) and flexed to about a 120 degree angle, do 8 to 16 Side Kicks with no bounce. The upper body should be upright and stable. Shorten the range of motion in the leg if the upper body moves. The knee flexion will increase the water's drag on the leg and increase the toning benefits. The knee joint should be consciously tightened by the students to avoid torque. The Side Lift Flex works abductors and adductors.

Side Press
The side press is a variation of the tricep extension and works the triceps and biceps. For Side Press Out begin with hands on hips and elbows out to the side. Turn palms away from the body (pronate) and press forearms out to the sides (extend elbows). For Side Press In return to beginning position from the extended Side Press Out. The press in concentrates on biceps while the press out concentrates on triceps.

Side Step
Begin with feet together and arms at sides. For the first count, step the right foot out to the right, keeping the toes pointed forward and allowing the knees to bend, while lifting both arms out to the sides (a reverse Press Down). Shift the body weight to the right foot and move the left foot next to the right foot's new position as arms lower for the second count. The body will be in beginning position about

– Sidekick Backward

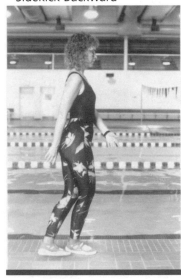

– Side Lift Flex

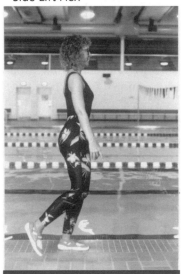

– Side Press

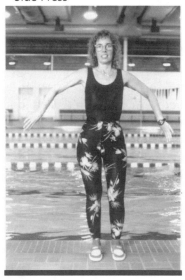

two feet to the right of the starting place. Repeat counts one and two 3 more times moving to the right. Side Step four to the left then by stepping the left foot out to the left and moving the right foot next to the left foot's new position. The Side Step works the abductors, adductors, deltoids and lattisimus dorsi. The arms can be straight or elbows can be flexed up to a 90 degree angle. Straight or slightly flexed arms will provide to highest intensity. Complete flexion will provide the lowest intensity.

Side Touch
See Touch Side

Side Train
Begin with feet together. For the first count, step the right foot out to the right side and shift the body weight to that leg by lifting the left foot up from beginning position. For the second count, step the left foot back to beginning position and shift the body weight to that leg by lifting the right foot up. Step the right foot back to beginning position for the third count and shift the body weight to that leg by lifting the left foot up from beginning position. For the fourth count, step the left foot back to beginning position. This is one Side Train Right. Repeat counts one through four 3 or 7 more times. Reverse for four or

eight Side Trains Left. The Side Train works abductors and adductors. A Lateral Push to the left as the right foot steps right during the Side Train Right and a Lateral Push to the right as the left foot steps left during the Side Train Left can be used. A reverse Press Down with elbows flexed or arms straight can also be used with the lift coming during the step to the right during the Side Train Right and during the step to the left during the Side Train Left.

Sidebend
Begin with feet in stride position, knees slightly flexed, hips tucked under and abdominals contracted. While bending sideways at the waist, tilt the upper torso toward the right (lateral

spinal flexion right). This a sidebend right. Repeat left for sidebend left. The sidebend works obliques. Participants should be cautioned to bend to the side only, not forward or back during the sidebend. The sidebend is a much smaller move than participants expect it to be. Emphasis should be put on the small range of motion that will be experienced.

Ski Bounce
Begin with feet in stride position. Bounce both feet together to the right and then bounce both feet together to the left as if shussing down a ski hill. This move can work quadriceps and hamstrings if done with a concentration on flexing and extending the knees. It can work

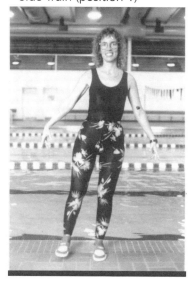

– Side Train (position 1)

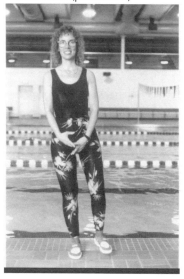

– Side Train (position 2)

obliques if done with concentration on the movement coming from the waist while keeping the upper torso stable. Tricep extensions back work well with the Ski Bounce.

Slide

The slide is a bouncing sidestep. It moves laterally to the right and then to the left. Begin in stride position. Step the right foot to the right side for the first count. Move the left leg to the right, stepping it next to the right while the right foot lifts off the pool bottom for the second count. Repeat counts one and two 3 to 7 times moving to the right. Step the left foot to the left for the first count on slide left. Move the right leg to the left, stepping it next to the left while the left leg lifts up off the pool bottom for the second count. Repeat counts one and two 3 to 7 times moving to the left. This is one full set of slides. The slide works adductors and abductors. Press Down arms work well with the slide.

Spider Crawl

Begin in a "spiderman" position on pool edge. Crawl or shuffle down the pool wall in one direction and switch direction. Feet should remain in contact with pool wall and hands should remain palms down on edge of pool. The more frequently direction is changed, the higher the intensity of the move.

Stroke

Begin with left hand on hip and right hand extended laterally to the left with palm facing forward. Push the right hand to the right just below the water's surface until the body has to pivot right as the right arms reaches slightly behind the body on the right side. Repeat with the left arm beginning on the right, and with the palm catching the water, push it to the left. This move works pectorals, deltoids, rhomboids and trapezius. For a faster pace, shorten the range of motion.

Swing Twist

Begin with feet in stride position. Bounce both feet (in place) to turn the toes of both feet to the right for the first count. This is a Swing Twist Right. Bounce both feet (in place) to turn the

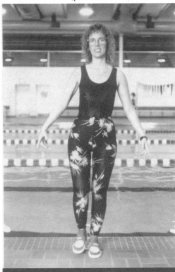
– Side Train (position 3)

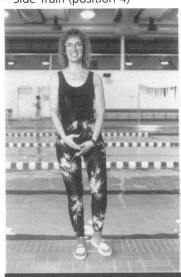
– Side Train (position 4)

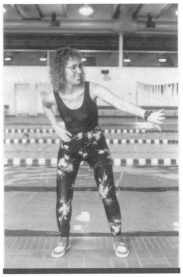
– Stroke

toes of both feet to the left for the second count. This is a Swing Twist Left. The entire move to both sides is one set of Swing Twists. During the Swing Twist Right both arms should push laterally to the left and during the Swing Twist Left the arms should push to the right. The Swing Twist works the obliques. This move can be varied by moving it forward and back or right and left or by turning it in a circle.

Swing Twist Doubles

Begin with feet in stride position. Bounce both feet (in place) to turn the toes of both feet to the right for the first count. Bounce once in that position for the second count. Bounce both feet (in place) to turn the toes of both feet to the left for the

third count. Bounce once in that position for the fourth count. This is one set of Swing Twist Doubles. This move works the obliques and can be varied like the Swing Twist.

Swing Twist in Three

The Swing Twist in Three begins with one set of Swing Twists for counts one and two. Counts three and four are Swing Twist Doubles right. Counts five and six are Swing Twists left and right. Counts seven and eight are Swing Twist Doubles left. The toes turn: Right, Left, Right, Right, Left, Right, Left, Left. This move works the obliques and can be varied like the Swing Twist.

Swing Twist with Back Toes Down

Begin doing a Swing Twist as described in Swing Twist. As the body twists right, the toes of the left foot (back foot) point down (plantar flex) toward the pool bottom. During the Swing Twist Left the toes of the back foot (right) point down toward the pool bottom. Pointing the "back" toes down during the Swing Twist adds gluteal work to the move, which ordinarily works the obliques. The "toes down" can be used during the Swing Twist, Swing Twist Doubles, and Swing Twist in Three.

Swing Twist with Front Toes Up

Begin doing a Swing Twist as described in Swing Twist. During the Swing Twist Right the toes of the front foot (right) point up toward the body (dorsiflex). During the Swing Twist Left the toes of the front foot (left) point up toward the body. The Swing Twist with Front Toes Up works obliques and tibialis anterior. The "toes up" can be used during the Swing Twist, Swing Twist Doubles, and Swing Twist in Three.

Swish

Begin in stride position with toes pointed slightly out (slight external hip rotation) and arms extended laterally (abducted) to just beneath the water surface.

– Swing Twist

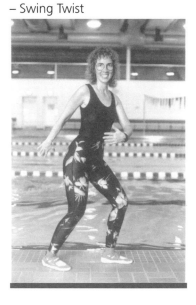

– Swing Twist with Back Toes Down

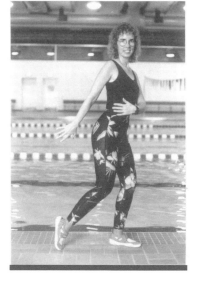

(Elbows are straight and arms are straight out to the sides). Rotate the spine (twist) to the right so that the right hand moves back about 6 to 12 inches and the left hand moves forward about 6 to 12 inches. Return to beginning position and then twist to the left so arms move 6 to 12 inches in the opposite direction. The body should not move from the hips down. Students will think this move is an arm movement...it is not. The arms stay in the same place in relation to the torso. The movement comes from the waist. The twisting at the waist causes the arms to move. The Swish works obliques. Students who are unable to accomplish this move without moving the lower body should pivot to the right during

the Swish right and visa versa. This will protect the knee joint.

Touch Back
Begin with feet in stride position. Touch the toes of the right foot back on the pool bottom for the first count. Return to beginning position for the second count. Touch the toes of the left foot back on the pool bottom for the third count. Return the left foot to beginning position for the fourth count. The right arm swings forward and the left arm swings back as the toes of the right foot touch back. Back touches can be done in series or four or eight right before changing to the left leg. They can also be done alternately as described above or in threes (RLRR, LRLL). Back touches work the

gluteals and iliopsoas.

Touch Forward
Begin with feet in stride position. For the first count, touch the toes of the right foot forward on the pool bottom. This will cause slight hip flexion. Left arm swings forward and right arm swings back as the toes on the right foot touch forward. Return to beginning position for the second count. Repeat counts one and two with the left leg for counts three and four. Forward touches can be done four or eight with the right foot before changing to using the left foot, or can be done alternately as described. Forward touches work the gluteals and iliopsoas.

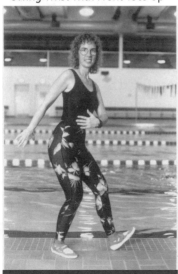

– Swing Twist with Front Toes Up

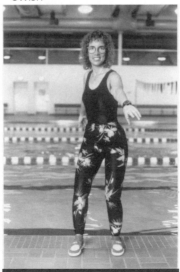

– Swish

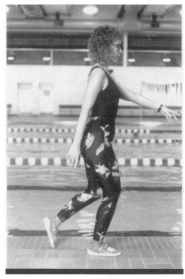

– Touch Back

Touch Side

Begin with feet together. Touch the toes of the right foot to the right side for the first count. Return to beginning position for the second count. Touch the toes of the left foot to the pool bottom on the left side for the third count. Return to beginning position for the fourth count. This is one set of Touch Side also called Side Touch. Side touches can be done "slow" with feet bouncing together between each touch as described above, or "fast" in a rocking type movement with the right foot returning to beginning position as the left foot is touching to the left and vice versa. Armswings side work well with Side Touches. Side touches can be done in a series or four or eight with the right foot before changing to using the left foot. Side touches work adductors and abductors.

Touch-Up

Side touch with the right foot while bouncing once on the left foot for the first count. Crossing kneelift with the right foot while bouncing once on the left foot for the second count. Repeat counts one and two three times before changing to the left foot. Side touch with the left foot while bouncing once on the left foot for the first count. Crossing kneelift with the left leg while bouncing once on the right foot for the second count.

Repeat counts one and two three more times with the left leg. This is one full set of touch ups. Since it is not recommended to bounce more than eight times

– Touch-Up (position 1)

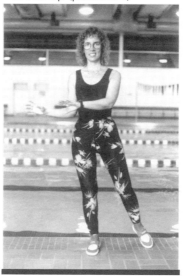

–Touch-Up (position 2)

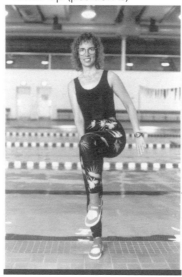

successively on one foot, no more than four touch ups should be done on one foot before changing to the other, unless weight is equally displaced between both legs during the side touch. Touch ups work iliopsoas, gluteals and abductors. Tricep extensions pressing back as the knee comes up work well with touch ups.

Trapezius Stretch

With fingers interlaced in front of the body at shoulder height, turn palms outward as arms are extended forward until a stretch is felt in the upper back. Trapezius can be stretched further by doing a neck stretch with right ear leaning toward right shoulder and the left ear leaning toward left shoulder and then chin relaxed and down on chest. An

– Trapezius Stretch

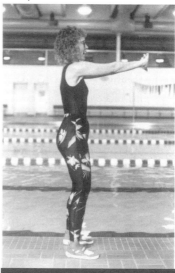

alternative trapezius stretch can be done by placing both hands on either side of the neck. Tilt the head forward and down.

Tricep Extension

Tricep extensions are generally the reverse of bicep curls but with palms facing the other way (pronated). Tricep extensions "back" begin with elbows flexed at about a 90 degree angle. Forearms are next to waist and elbows are about three to six inches back from the body. Arms (shoulders) are slightly hyperextended. In this position forearms should be pressed back through the water (elbow extension). Tricep extensions "out" begin in the same position but palms are facing out (away from the body). To accomplish the tricep extension forearms should be pressed out through the water. Tricep extensions "forward" begin with elbows next to the waist and completely flexed. They are accomplished by extending the elbow or pressing the palms down to the sides of the thighs. They work the triceps and biceps.

Tricep Stretch

With arms overhead, hold the elbow of the right arm with the left hand. Gently pull the right elbow to the left behind the head, creating a stretch in the tricep. To increase the stretch, bend the elbow of the right arm.

This also stretches the latissimus dorsi. Reverse for left.

Tuck Jump

Begin with feet in stride position

– Tricep Extension Back

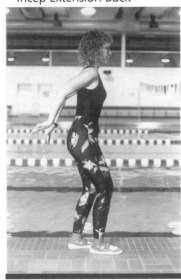

– Tricep Extension Forward

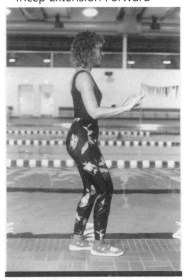

and arms extended laterally just below the water surface. Pull both knees up to the chest while pressing arms down through the water to under the knees. Tuck

– Tricep Extension Out

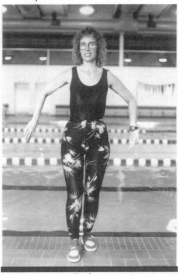

– Tricep Stretch

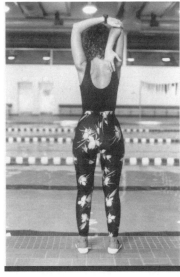

jumps work iliopsoas and gluteals. Abdominal muscles should be contracted during the tuck jump.

Twist

Begin with feet in wide stride position, knees slightly flexed, hips tucked under, abdominals tightened and ribs lifted. While keeping the toes, knees and hips pointed forward, twist the upper torso toward the right (spinal rotation right). This is the first count of twist. Return to beginning position for the second count. Twist the torso to the left for the third count and return to beginning position for the fourth count. This is one set of twist. The twist works obliques. The twist can be varied to protect the integrity of the

knee joint by pivoting the feet, knees and hips in the same direction as the twist.

Two Step

Two step is simply two side steps right followed by two side steps left. For a complete description, see Side Step.

Waist Curls

Waist curls are bicep curls with elbows staying close to the waist. They work the biceps and triceps. They can be done "forward" with the forearm forward moving up and down, they can be done "in" with the forearm across the body moving up and down and they can be done "out" with the forearms out to the sides moving up and down. The palm, in all waist curls, is facing up (supinated).

Waterpull

Begin with both arms extended laterally to the left, then pull the elbows in toward the waist. Palms are facing forward. This is the beginning position. Push both arms through the water to the right and then to the left. The range of motion will be short because of the flexed position of the elbows. Lowering the arms deeper into the water and then bringing them back to the surface will increase the interest and intensity of this move. This move works biceps and triceps but can be modified to

work pectorals, deltoids, rhomboids and trapezius by extending the elbows. It is often done without any foot movement for upper body toning but Rock Side to Side can work well with it.

Wind-Up and Present

Begin with arms extended laterally with palms down. With elbow extended so that arm is straight, press the right arm down in front of body and continue moving it left and up until it is parallel with the left arm. This is the "windup" portion of the move. Turn palm of right arm out and push across, just below the water's surface, to beginning position. This is the "present" portion of the move. Continue with several using the right arm and then switching to

– Tuck Jump

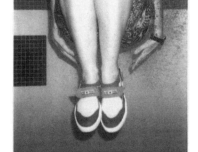

– Waterpull

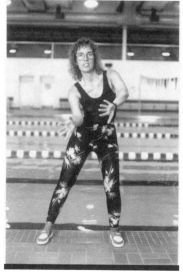

the left or alternate using the right and left arms. Pectorals, deltoids, trapezius and rhomboids are all involved in Windup and Present. To involve obliques, keep the lower body stationary with the feet in a wide stance, with feet and toes pointed slightly outwards. If obliques are not desired in the move, keep the knee joint safe by pivoting the feet and knees in the same direction.

– Wind-Up and Present (position 1)

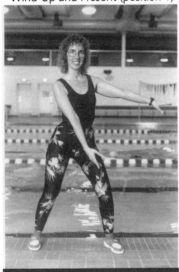

– Wind-Up and Present (position 2)

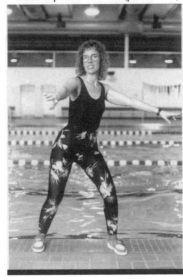

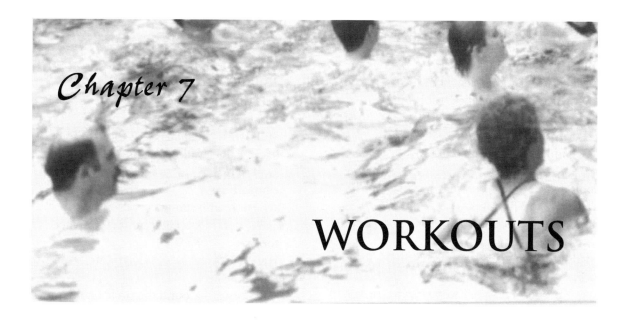

Chapter 7

WORKOUTS

Aqua Strength Training

Thermal Warm-Up

Do the following for 1 minute each:

A. Jog or walk, forward and back (usually 8 or 16 jogs forward and 8 or 16 jogs backward, depending on pool size)

B. Continue jogging or walking, bending the knee and pulling the heel back to the buttock

C. Continue jogging or walking, using high kneelifts

D. Change to walking or jogging sideways (8 or 16 to the right, 8 or 16 to the left)

E. Jumping jacks with arms beneath the water surface

Prestretch

Hold the following stretches for 10 to 15 seconds each:

A. Quadriceps right, quadriceps left

B. Hamstring right, hamstring left

C. Calf right, calf left

D. Hip flexor right, hip flexor left

E. Pectorals

F. Trapezius

Weight Training

1. Do the following for 90 seconds each with force:

A. Bicep curls up

B. Tricep extensions down

C. Pectoral presses (elbow press forward) with elbows bent

D. Trapezius/rhomboid pulls (elbow press back) with elbows bent

E. Latissimus dorsi presses (press down behind)

F. Deltoid lifts

2. Do the following with the right leg for 90 seconds each with force; then repeat with the left leg:
   A. Knee flexion (mule kick)
   B. Hip flexion (kick forward)
   C. Hip abduction (side lift)
   D. Knee extension (flick kick)
   E. Hip extension (back kick)
   F. Hip adduction (cross kick)
   G. Hip circumduction (circles)

Cooldown
Walk for 2 to 3 minutes.

Poststretch
Do the following stretches for 20 to 30 seconds each:
   A. Knee flexion (quadricep stretch), right and left
   B. Hip flexion (gluteal stretch), right and left
   C. Hip abduction (abductor stretch), right and left
   D. Knee extension (hamstring stretch), right and left
   E. Hip extension (iliopsoas stretch), right and left
   F. Hip adduction (adductor stretch), right and left
   G. Bicep stretch
   H. Tricep stretch, right and left
   I. Pectoral stretch
   J. Trapezius stretch
   K. Deltoid (medial) stretch, right and left

Water Walking

Wearing shoes is recommended.

Thermal Warm-Up
Do the following for 45 seconds each:
   A. Walk with small steps, 12 forward and 12 back, using walking arms (the right arm swings forward as the left leg steps forward), elbows bent
   B. Repeat A with shoulder rolls
   C. Walk forward in a circle, rolling from heel to toe
   D. Walk backward in a circle, rolling from the toe to the heel
   E. Walk forward around the circle on the toes
   F. Walk backward around the circle on the heels
   G. Do toe circles for 20 seconds with the right foot and 20 seconds with the left foot

Prestretch
   A. Calf stretch, right and left (15 seconds each)
   B. Walk forward around the circle; push both arms forward for trapezius/rhomboid stretch (20 seconds)
   C. Walk backward around the circle, using a shoulder blade pinch to stretch the pectorals (20 seconds)
   D. Walk forward to the right corner; walk back using mule kicks (20 seconds)
   E. Repeat D to the left corner and back (20 seconds)
   F. Quadricep stretch, right and left (15 seconds each)
   G. Hip flexor stretch, right and left (15 seconds each)
   H. Hamstring stretch, right and left (15 seconds each)

I. Calf stretch, right and left (15 seconds each)
J. Walk forward and back using sidebends (30 seconds)

Cardiovascular Warm-Up

1. Do the following in circle formation for 45 seconds each:
    A. Moving forward, take exaggerated, long strides, keeping the knees bent. Add jogging arms, with the hands cupped.
    B. Keep the knees bent and move double time with smaller steps. Change the arms to punching.
    C. Repeat A and B.

2. Face the center of the circle, and do the following for 45 seconds each:
    A. Walk sideways using lateral push arms. Move 8 to the right and 8 to the left repeatedly until the time allotment is finished.
    B. Walk sideways using deltoid lift arms. Move 8 to the right and 8 to the left repeatedly until the time allotment is finished.
    C. Walk in and out of the circle using breaststroke and backstroke arms.
    D. Add high knees to 2C and continue.
    E. Straighten the legs to a goose step, moving in and out of the circle.
    F. Repeat B, C, D, and E.

Aerobics

The Aerobics portion is 15 minutes. Do the following exercises for 45 seconds each:

Group 1—In scatter formation:
A. Walk forward on the toes (bent elbow, walking arms); walk back on the heels.
B. Walk sideways using sidekicks. Move 8 to the right and 8 to the left repeatedly until the time allotment is finished.
C. Walk forward and back using mule kicks.

Group 2—In scatter formation:
A. Walk in a square with the knees and toes pointed somewhat out.
B. Repeat A, moving backward.
C. Walk forward and back, using side bends.
D. Walk, leaning forward while moving forward and leaning back while moving back.

Group 3—In circle formation:
A. Walk forward into the circle, using high knees.
B. Continue with high knees, but cross the right foot over the left and lower the right as the step is taken (strut).
C. Walk backward around the circle, crossing the right foot behind the left and the left behind the right.

Group 4—In circle formation:
A. Walk around the circle, using high knees.
B. Continue walking around the circle, but change to a goose step.
C. Continue walking around the circle, but change to a flick kick.
D. Repeat A through C, moving backward around the circle.

Group 5—In circle formation:
A. Walk around the circle, contracting and releasing the abdominals.
B. Walk backward, using diagonal kicks.
C. Move forward, using sidekicks and stepping across.
D. Turn around and go back (again, facing forward), using sidekicks and stepping behind.

Cooldown

Do the following in scatter formation for 1 minute each:

A. Walk 4 low and 4 high (2 sets forward and 2 sets back).
B. Walk 4 fast and 8 slow, forward and back.
C. Walk sideways, 2 slow and 4 fast (2 sets right, 2 sets left).
D. Over and present.
E. Walk forward and back, using shoulder rolls.

Upper-Body Toning

Do the following for 45 seconds each (3-1/2 minutes total):

A. Elbow press
B. Elbow press back
C. Bicep curls
D. Tricep extensions
E. Push across

Edge-of-Pool Toning

Do the following for 1 minute each:

A. Side lifts—Do 10 with the force on the lift out and 10 with the force on the return in. Repeat.
B. Knee flexion (mule kick)—Do 10 with the force on pulling the heel back and 10 with the force on straightening the leg.
C. Knee swings
D. Turn the other side to the pool edge and repeat with the other leg.

Stretch

Hold each for 30 seconds (5 minutes total):

A. Quadricep stretch, right and left
B. Calf stretch, right and left
C. Hamstring stretch, right and left
D. Pectoral stretch
E. Iliopsoas stretch, right and left
F. Back stretch, push forward
G. Adductor stretch, right and left

Aerobics

Do the following workout 3 times on nonconsecutive days:

Thermal Warm-Up

Do the following for 1 minute each (4 minutes total):

A. Hoedowns
B. Jazz kicks
C. Sidekicks
D. Cross kicks

Stretch

Do the following for 15 seconds each (3 minutes total):

A. Quadricep stretch, right and left
B. Calf stretch, right and left
C. Hamstring stretch, right and left
D. Pectoral stretch
E. Iliopsoas stretch, right and left
F. Back stretch
G. Adductor stretch, right and left

Cardiovascular Warm-Up

Do the following for five minutes total:

A. Hopscotch, 1 minute
B. Sidekicks (repeat 4 left, 4 right), 1 minute
C. Forward kicks, slow and fast, 2 minutes
D. Kneelifts fast, 1 minute

Aerobics

Do each of the following for 45 seconds (15 minutes total):

Group 1
  Jumping jacks
  Jumping jacks crossing
  Forward kicks fast
  Forward kicks slow

Workouts

Group 2
  Sidekicks
  Mule kicks fast
  Mule kicks doubles
  Flick kicks (repeat 8 left, 8 right)
  Jazzkicks
Group 3
  Diagonal kicks fast
  Diagonal kicks slow
  Diagonal kicks slow (repeat 4 left, 4 right)
  Jog forward slow and backward fast
  Jumping jacks, slow and fast
Group 4
  Scissors
  Scissors with front toes up
  Scissors with back toes down
  Jog tilt (8 leaning forward, 8 leaning backward)
  Kneelifts

Cooldown

Do the following for 1 minute each (3 minutes total):
  A. Jog in place, fast and slow
  B. Rock from side to side
  C. Mule kicks

Upper-Body Toning

Do the following for 45 seconds each (3-1/2 minutes total):
  A. Elbow press
  B. Elbow press back
  C. Bicep curls
  D. Tricep extensions
  E. Push across

Edge-of-Pool Toning

Do the following for 1 minute each:
  A. Side lifts—Do 10 with the force on the lift out and 10 with the force on the return in. Repeat.
  B. Knee flexion (mule kick)—Do 10 with the force on pulling the heel back and 10 with the force on straightening the leg.
  C. Knee swings
  D. Turn the other side to the pool edge and repeat with the other leg.

Stretch

Hold each for 30 seconds (5 minutes total):
  A. Quadricep stretch, right and left
  B. Calf stretch, right and left
  C. Hamstring stretch, right and left
  D. Pectoral stretch
  E. Iliopsoas stretch, right and left
  F. Back stretch, push forward
  G. Adductor stretch, right and left

Toning

Thermal Warm-Up

A. Walk fast in a big circle, moving clockwise, for 30 seconds.

B. Move back around the circle for 30 seconds.

C. Walk fast with high knees, moving counter-clockwise, for 30 seconds.

D. Back up for 30 seconds.

E. Walk sideways, moving right 8 to 10 steps and then left 8 to 10 steps, for 1 minute

F. Walk with sidebends around the circle for 30 seconds.

G. Back up with sidebends for 30 seconds.

H. Walk around the circle counterclockwise, kicking the heel toward the buttocks, for 30 seconds.

I. Back up, kicking the heel toward the buttocks, for 30 seconds.

J. Walk around the circle on the heels for 30 seconds.

K. Back up around the circle on the heels for 30 seconds.

Prestretch

Hold each of the following for 15 to 20 seconds:

A. Calf stretch, right and left

B. Iliopsoas stretch, right and left

C. Hamstring stretch, right and left

D. Quadricep stretch, right and left

E. Adductor stretch, right and left

F. Pectoral stretch

G. Back stretch

Toning

At the pool edge, do each of the following for 24 repetitions or 1 minute. Do those exercises that are repeated on the right and left sides for 1 minute on each side.

A. Bicep curls, right and left

B. Mule kicks, right and left

C. Tricep extensions, right and left

D. Flick kicks, right and left

E. Swing the arms, forward and backward (with emphasis on arm extension or pull back)

F. Kickswing, right and left (with emphasis on hip extension)

G. Deltoid lift (both arms together)

H. Side lifts, right and left (hip abduction)

I. Press down (both arms together)

J. Cross kicks, right and left

K. Elbow press forward

L. Abdominal crunches

M. Elbow press back

N. Kick swing, right and left (with emphasis on hip flexion or kick)

O. Swing the arms together, forward and backward (with emphasis on swing forward or shoulder flexion)

P. Punch across (alternating arms)

Cooldown and Poststretch

A. Do A and B from Warm-Up

B. Bicep stretch, 15 to 20 seconds

C. Trapezius stretch, 15 to 20 seconds

D. Do C and D from Warm-Up

E. Quadricep stretch, right and left

F. Hip flexor stretch, right and left

F. Do E from Warm-Up with tricep stretch, right and left, and neck stretch, right and left

G. Do F and G from Warm-Up

H. Abductor stretch, right and left

I. Adductor stretch, right and left

J. Do H and I from Warm-Up

K. Hamstring stretch, right and left

L. Calf stretch, right and left

M. Back stretch

Flexibility

Warm-Up

Do the following in circle formation:

A. Walk fast, moving clockwise, for 30 seconds.

B. Back up for 30 seconds.

C. Walk fast with high knees, moving counter-clockwise, for 30 seconds.

D. Back up for 30 seconds.

E. Walk sideways, moving 8 to 10 steps to the right and 8 to 10 steps to the left, for 1 minute.

F. Walk forward with sidebends around the circle for 30 seconds.

G. Back up with sidebends.

H. Walk, kicking the heels toward the buttocks, moving counterclockwise, for 30 seconds.

I. Back up, kicking the heels toward the buttocks, for 30 seconds.

Arms

Use the following arm movements with A through I above:

A. Tricep extensions

B. Bicep curls

C. Punching the opposite arm forward

D. Backstrokes

E. Deltoid lifts

F & G. Press Downs

H & I. Swing the corresponding arm forward and up and the opposite arm

Flexibility

Upper Body—Jog or walk while doing the following stretches to keep body temperature at a comfortable level. If the body becomes chilled and muscles tighten, stop stretching and go through the Warm-Up phase more vigorously until body temperature is warm enough for comfortable, relaxed stretching.

Hold each of the following for 20 to 30 seconds:

A. Push both arms up, lifting from the ribs

B. Trapezius stretch

C. Pectoral stretch

D. Tricep stretch, right and left

E. Bicep stretch

F. Neck stretch, right and left

G. Walk with shoulder rolls

Lower Body—Hold each of the following stretches for 30 seconds:

A. Do C and D from the Warm-Up

B. Iliopsoas stretch, right and left

C. Gluteal stretch, right and left

D. Do E from the Warm-Up

E. Adductor stretch, right and left

F. Abductor stretch, right and left

G. Do F and G from the Warm-Up

H. Oblique stretch, right and left

I. Do H and I from the Warm-Up

J. Quadricep stretch, right and left

K. Hamstring stretch, right and left

L. Walk forward on the toes and back on the heels for 1 minute

M. Calf stretch, right and left

N. Tibialis anterior stretch, right and left

O. Back stretch

P. Abdominal stretch

Cooldown

Walk slowly around the pool for 3 minutes.

Circuit Training

Thermal Warm-Up

Do each of the following for 1 minute:

- A. Jumping jacks and sidekicks
- B. Kneelifts moving forward, crosskicks back
- C. Heelhits, front and back
- D. Kneeswing combo in place, up and back (4 right, 4 left), cross (4 right, 4 left)

Prestretch

Do each of the following for 10 to15 seconds:

- A. Quadricep stretch, right and left
- B. Iliopsoas stretch, right and left
- C. Hamstring stretch, right and left
- D. Scissors with pectoral stretch
- E. Calf stretch, right and left
- F. Back stretch

Cardiovascular Warm-Up

Do each of the following for 1 minute:

- A. Kicks, slow and fast
- B. Jumping jacks crossing
- C. Slides (16 right, 16 left)
- D. Ski bounces
- E. Swing twists in 3

Aerobics

For each of the following, spend 1 minute doing each station movement and 2 minutes doing each aerobics segment:

First station—Elbow press, forward and back

Aerobics—Jog forward, heelhits back (any mix); add jazzkick

Second station—Mule kicks, right leg

Aerobics—Swing twist singles and doubles (any mix); vary with the toes of the back foot down and the toes of the front foot up; move forward and back and side to side

Third station—Bicep curls, tricep extensions

Aerobics—Side steps and scissors (any mix)

Fourth station—Mule kicks, left leg

Aerobics—Bounce square; add scissors moving forward, jumping jacks back

Fifth station—Kickswings, right leg

Aerobics—Sidekicks, 4 right and 4 left

Sixth station—Deltoid lifts, press down

Aerobics—Jump bounce, 4 forward and 4 back; add kicks, slow and fast

Seventh station—Kickswings, left leg

Aerobics—Slide; add kicks forward, ski bounces back

Eighth station—Side leglifts, right leg

Aerobics—Mule kicks, slow and fast; add jumping jacks and jumping jacks crossing

Ninth station—Side leglifts, left leg

Aerobics—Back kicks, slow and fast; add back kicks forward, kneelifts back

Tenth station—Abdominal crunches

Aerobics—Kicks and fling kicks; add flings and heelhits front

Eleventh station—Crosskicks, right leg

Aerobics—Rockinghorse 7 and up; add tuck jumps

Twelfth station—Crosskicks, left leg

Aerobics—Kneelifts forward, heel hits back, slow and fast; add rocking side to side

Thirteenth station—Flick kicks, right leg

Aerobics—Jumping jacks square, 4 each direction (right, back, left, forward); add crossing kneelifts, 4 right and 4 left

Fourteenth station—Flick kicks, left leg

Aerobics—Scissors and ski bounces

Cooldown and Flexibility

Do the following and hold the stretches for 20 to 30 seconds each:

- A. Swing twists with flag arms
- B. Walk 8 forward, kick, walk 8 back; repeat 3 times

C. Bounce 8 times

D. Adductor stretch, right and left

E. Side step with tricep stretch

F. Side step with neck stretch

G. Side step with shoulder stretch

H. Swing twist 16 times

I. Iliopsoas stretch, right and left

J. Kneeswing combo, 4 sets

K. Hamstring stretch, right and left

L. Pectoral stretch

M. Corner jazzkick 32 times

N. Quadricep stretch, right and left

O. Back stretch

P. Heel jacks 32 times

Q. Calf stretch, right and left

R. Push both arms up

Sport Specific

Thermal Warm-Up

Do each of the following for 1 minute:

A. Walk with long, exertive strides, forward and back.

B. Jog forward and back, with hçûh knees. Use bicep curls and tricep extensions.

C. Sidestep 8 to 10 steps to the right and 8 to 10 steps to the left. Use deltoid lift and press down arms.

D. Jog in place, with heels kicking up and back (like mule kicks). Use elbow press forward and back.

Prestretch

Hold each of the following for 10 to 15 seconds:

A. Calf stretch, right and left

B. Iliopsoas stretch, right and left

C. Hamstring stretch, right and left

D. Back stretch

Cardiovascular Warm-Up

Do the following combination movements/ stretches:

A. Do 16 sidesteps to the right while doing a tricep stretch right.

B. Do 16 sidesteps to the left while doing a tricep stretch left.

C. Repeat A and B.

D. Do 32 jumping jacks while doing a pectoral stretch.

E. Do 32 jumping jacks while doing a deltoid lift and press down.

F. Do 8 jumping jacks moving forward and 8 moving back; repeat this sequence (8 up, 8 back) 4 times.

G. Do 32 scissors.

Aerobics

Balance and Coordination

A. Do 32 ski bounces while doing tricep extensions.

B. Do 16 ski bounces moving forward and 16 moving back; repeat this sequence (16 up, 16 back) 4 times.

C. Do 32 ski bounces in place with the right foot only.

D. Repeat C with the left leg.

E. Bounce 4 times moving sideways to the right and 4 times moving sideways to the left; add the lateral press arm movement. Repeat this sequence (4 right, 4 left) 4 times.

F. Repeat E using only the right foot.

G. Repeat E using only the left foot.

H. Bounce 16 times in a square, such that the first bounce makes the right corner of the square (bounce right, back, left, forward to make the square). Bounce another 16, such that the first bounce makes the left corner of the square (bounce left, back, right, forward). Add the jump rope arm movement.

I. Repeat H using the right leg only.

J. Repeat H using the left leg only.

Intervals

A. Do scissors at moderate intensity for 30 seconds; swing the arms alternately forward and back.

B. Do scissors at high intensity for 30 seconds. Use more power, lengthen the stride, use a larger range of motion with the arms, and push up off the pool bottom with more effort.

C. Repeat A and B 3 more times.

Power

A. Do tuck jumps, 8 moving forward and 8 moving back. Do the sequence (8 forward, 8 back) covering a moderate amount of distance and twice covering the largest distance possible.

B. Do jump bounces, 1 forward and 1 back; do 16 sets.

C. Do 3 small bounces and 1 big jump, covering a maximum distance on the big jump. Move 4 forward and 4 back; repeat this sequence (4 moving forward, 4 moving back) 4 times.

D. Run with long strides to form a circle; move forward around the circle for 2 minutes.

Intervals

A. Do jumping jacks at moderate intensity for 30 seconds.

B. Do jumping jack jumps at high intensity for 30 seconds.

C. Repeat A and B 3 more times.

Sport Stations—Spend 1 minute each at 4 different stations of your choice:

A. Baseball bats

B. Tennis racquets

C. Power mule kick drills

D. Basketball jumps

E. Run and hurdle

F. Sprinting

G. Run and long jump

H. Golf clubs

Cooldown and Flexibility

A. Walk for 2 minutes with varied strides.

B. Sidestep 16 to the right while doing a shoulder stretch right.

C. Sidestep 16 to the left while doing a shoulder stretch left.

D. Sidestep 16 to the right while doing a tricep stretch right.

E. Sidestep 16 to the left while doing a tricep stretch left.

F. Calf stretch, right and left, 15 seconds each

G. Do 24 scissors.

H. Iliopsoas stretch, right and left, 15 seconds each

I. Hamstring stretch, right and left, 15 seconds each

J. Do 24 jumping jacks.

K. Back stretch, 15 seconds

L. Pectoral stretch, 15 seconds

M. Repeat A.

Deep Water:
Using Flotation Vests or Belts

Thermal Warm-Up

Do each of the following for 1 minute:

A. Jog forward at moderate intensity, using tricep extensions.

B. Jog backward at moderate intensity, using bicep curls.

C. Do jumping jacks with deltoid lifts and press downs.

D. Do scissors, with arms alternately swinging forward and backward.

Prestretch

Do each of the following for 10 to 15 seconds:

A. Hamstring stretch, right and left

B. Quadricep stretch, right and left

C. Iliopsoas stretch, right and left

D. Pectoral stretch

E. Back stretch

F. Calf stretch, right and left (at the edge of the pool, pressing the foot of the leg to be stretched against the pool wall)

Cardiovascular Warm-Up

Do each of the following for 1 minute:

A. Jog with high knees, staying in place.

B. Jog with high knees, moving forward by using breaststroke arms.

C. Jog with high knees, moving backward by using backstroke arms.

D. Jog with heels kicking up and back (mule kick), staying in place.

E. Repeat D, moving forward using breaststroke arms. (The abdominals must be contracted, and no hip flexion should occur.)

F. Repeat D, moving backward using backstroke arms.

Aerobics

1. Do each of the following for 1 minute:
   A. Scissors at moderate intensity, staying in place
   B. Scissors, moving forward by using crawl arms
   C. Scissor jumps, using enough force to push the body up and out of the water
   D. Scissors, moving backward by using single arms alternating the backstroke

2. Do each of the following:
   A. Scissor and jumping jack combo (1 scissor, 1 jumping jack); repeat for 1 minute
   B. Kneelifts in 3—4 sets in place and 4 sets moving forward; 4 sets in place and 4 sets moving backward
   C. Scissors—16 times each: toes pointed out, toes pointed down, toes pointed up. Repeat this sequence (16 out, 16 down, 16 up) twice.
   D. Mule kicks—16 moving forward, kneelifts, 16 moving backward; repeat this sequence (16 forward, kneelifts, 16 backward) 4 times.
   E. Scissors—16 with long, slow strides, 16 with short, fast strides; repeat this sequence (16 long, 16 short) twice.

3. Do each of the following for 1 minute:
   A. Jumping jacks, staying in place
   B. Jumping jacks, moving forward using breaststroke arms (the abdominals must be contracted, and hip hyperextension should not occur)
   C. Jumping jack jumps (the legs should close with enough force to push the body up and out of the water)
   D. Jumping jacks, moving backward using backstroke arms.
   E. Jumping jacks crossing
   F. Jumping jacks, alternating with toes pointed down and up

Cooldown

Do each of the following for 1 minute:
   A. Jog forward with mule kicks
   B. Jog backward with kneelifts
   C. Mule kicks in place
   D. Kneelifts in place
   E. Heel hits in front
   F. Heel hits behind

Toning and Flexibility

1. Work at the edge of the pool, with one side to the pool wall (work same side, right or left, for entire sequence). Repeat each movement 32 times; hold each stretch for 15 seconds.
   A. Side leg lift
   B. Adductor stretch
   C. Kickswing
   D. Iliopsoas stretch
   E. Side leg circles
   F. Abductor stretch
   G. Mule kicks
   H. Hamstring stretch

2. Switch sides, turning the other side to the pool wall. Repeat A through H. Again, repeat each movement 32 times; hold each stretch for 15 seconds.

3. Continue as follows:
   A. With the back to the pool edge, do elbow presses forward and back
   B. With the back still to the pool edge, do pectoral stretch
   C. Facing the pool edge, do deltoid lifts and press downs
   D. Back stretch
   E. Calf stretch, right and left (press the foot of the leg being stretched against the pool wall)

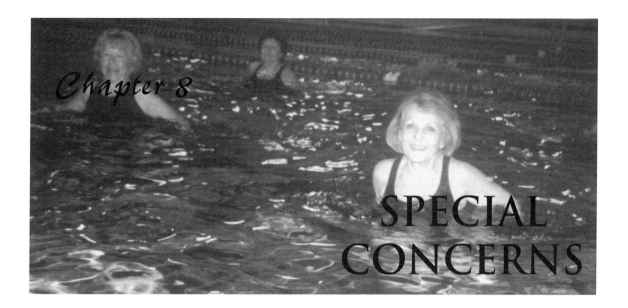

Chapter 8

SPECIAL CONCERNS

Because of the relative weightlessness of participants, water exercise is an excellent low-impact aerobic activity for people who have some physical difficulty. This makes water aerobics the exercise of choice for those millions of people who are overweight or pregnant; who suffer from arthritis, other joint problems, or back or knee pain; or who need rehabilitation or therapy after recent surgery or childbirth. In all of these cases, the instructor must be certain to lead participants through an extended warm-up phase. Full, controlled movements should be substituted for choppy, jerky ones. Progressive overload should be extremely gradual.

Basic Precautions

Health History and Physician's Approval

Although water exercise is one of the safest ways to work out, participants should be advised that this is an exertive program. All participants should inform their physicians of their intention to take part in aquatic exercise. An exerciser with a history of any type of medical problem should obtain his or her physician's approval along with possible suggestions to adapt the program to his or her individual needs.

Overexertion

If exercisers experience pain during any workout, they should be advised to stop exercising, walk slowly in place, and inform their instructor. Instructors should watch for participants who display any of the following signs of overexertion:

- nausea
- extreme weakness
- profuse sweating
- red face
- breathlessness
- excessive fatigue
- chest pain or discomfort
- lightheadedness or dizziness
- focused musculoskeletal discomfort
- ataxic (unsteady) gait
- confusion

Instructors need to be prepared to handle minor and major medical emergencies. CPR, first aid, and emergency water rescue certification are strongly recommended.

Aquatic exercise instructors should understand the sources of fatigue so that the symptoms listed above can be eliminated.

Hyperthermia

Hyperthermia is the overheating of the body, which can happen in warm water or areas with very little circulation. The participant will feel an overall loss of energy.

Glycogen Depletion

Glycogen depletion causes graduated and overall fatigue. Participants should keep the workout at low to moderate intensity for short periods and gradually overload to avoid glycogen depletion.

Musculoskeletal Fatigue

Musculoskeletal fatigue is often recognized by pain in a bone, joint, or muscle. Overdoing any one exercise movement can cause musculoskeletal fatigue.

Lactic Acid Accumulation

Lactic acid accumulation comes on relatively quickly and is usually focused in one particular muscle group. It can be avoided by shortening the duration and intensity of the workout and by varying the exercise.

Special Populations
Older Adults

Kenny Moore, Olympic marathon runner said, "You don't stop exercising because you grow old. You grow old because you stop exercising." The American Medical Association's Committee on Aging studied the phenomenon of aging and found that it is virtually impossible to discriminate between the effects of aging and the effects of inactivity. Exercise is the fountain of youth.

Programs should include stretching to improve or maintain range of motion and flexibility and exercises to improve general postural alignment. Regular exercise has been shown to increase joint flexibility and decrease joint pain in most adults.

The class format for an older adult program should follow that of the traditional aerobics class. The older adult may need to spend more warming up in order to release synovial fluid in the joints and deliver oxygen to the muscles. Everyone should be comfortably warm in the water before the vigorous, high-intensity workout begins. The intensity of the workout should be modified according to individual fitness levels. The program format should also include time for socializing while exercising, touching (some older adults who live alone no longer have anyone close enough to them to touch them), and working on balance or coordination activities.

Major muscle groups and fine-motor skills should be included in the programming. Exercise instructors often spend time working only major muscle groups. The older adult needs to also work the smaller muscles in the body to improve fine-motor skills. (Simply opening and closing the hands is an example of a fine-motor skill.)

Programs for older adults should use music from their era. Music such as Big Band, ragtime, and Broadway hits is enjoyable for older adults. They like the subtle rhythms from their time more than the pounding rhythms that are heard now. Avoid using excessively high volume with the music. Some older adult classes prefer not to have any music for background during their class, as it interferes with their hearing the instructor.

The older adult who is unfit should begin exercise at the low end of the target zone or perceived exertion chart. Heartrates will often be affected by medications. Progressive overload should be extremely gradual in terms of frequency, duration, and especially intensity.

Older adults tend to appreciate warmer water than younger adults and swimmers. If possible, water temperature in the 86- to 88-degree range is recommended.

Equipment that does not require excessive gripping is recommended, since joint problems and arthritis can be exacerbated by prolonged gripping. Aqua gloves seem to work exceptionally well. Other types of equipment can all be successful if they are used only for a portion of the class and in adherence to the concept of progressive overload.

Obese Individuals

Obesity is defined as being above 23% to 25% body fat for men and 30% to 33% percent body fat for women. The average body fat for men is approximately 15%, while the average for women is 25%.

Not only do modifications need to be made because of the amount of weight a participant is exercising with but also because obesity predisposes participants to other medical problems: diabetes, high cholesterol, high levels of LDL cholesterol, and a high risk of coronary artery disease and hypertension. The obese person is also predisposed to a greater likelihood of musculoskeletal injuries and overexertion. The cardiovascular demands of exercise are much greater for an obese person because of the mass needing to be moved and the great likelihood of atrophied muscles due to inactivity.

The obese often have poor coordination and balance, which will be alleviated somewhat by the water. Exercise patterns should be simple to follow. Some exercisers may prefer to hold onto the pool edge when first beginning class. In order to keep the impact as light as possible, the obese exerciser should move as deep in the water as possible without losing control of the motion. Deep water provides more buoyancy. Unfortunately, obese people are usually very buoyant also. Mov-

ing too deep in the water to lessen the impact can cause floundering, loss of control of the exercise, and panic. The instructor and students should work together to find a water depth that will allow students to exercise safely with as little impact as possible.

The obese person may want to wear cushioned aqua shoes to protect the bottoms of the feet from the abrasive pool. This will also aid in absorbing any impact during the program.

If the pool water, air temperature, or air humidity become high, obese participants will be at high risk for heat exhaustion. Because of their weight, they will have more difficulty dissipating heat. They are also more likely to experience hyperpnea and dyspnea (excessive or difficult breathing).

The format of the class for obese participants will be modified only slightly. The warm-up is the same as for a regular aerobics class, but the aerobic portion should be at a lower intensity and of a longer duration. The cooldown may need to be increased in duration to ensure proper relief. The toning can be eliminated if the elongated aerobic portion demands it.

The average aerobics water temperature (80 degrees to 84 degrees) seems comfortable for most obese participants. Water temperatures of 86 degrees and higher can trigger heat-stress syndromes.

Prenatal Women

Many theories have considered the effects of exercise on a pregnant woman and fetus. Research results have been limited, divergent, and seem somewhat inconclusive. Generally, studies show that healthy pregnant women experience very few negative effects from moderate exercise.

Many special considerations factor into a prenatal exercise program. The prenatal woman experiences postural changes that alter the center of gravity and weight gains that may lead to lordosis and often kyphosis.

Lordosis is an exaggerated anterior (forward) curvature of the lumbar spine (swayback), and kyphosis is an exaggerated posterior curvature of the thoracic spine (rounded shoulders, dowagers hump). The pregnant woman often compensates for the excess weight carried in her stomach by sticking her buttocks backward and her head forward.

Plasma volume increases during pregnancy, which can cause problems with circulation such as swelling, cramping, and supine hypotension. Weight increases can also increase the workload on the heart, respiratory system, and joints.

In 1994, the American College of Obstetricians and Gynecologists (ACOG) set guidelines for exercise safety during pregnancy. The guidelines included information on the following:

Frequency – Regular exercise, at least three times per week, is preferable to intermittent exercise.

Intensity – An intensity level of mild to moderate should be set. The pregnant woman should never exercise to exhaustion.

Mode – Exercises in the supine position should be eliminated after the fourth month of pregnancy. The Valsalva maneuver should not be used. Non-weight bearing exercises will minimize the risk of injury.

ACOG also stated that the pregnant women should augment heat dissipation with hydration, appropriate clothing and optimal environmental surroundings. Caloric intake should be adequate to meet the extra metabolic needs of an additional 300 kilocalories per day. Morphological changes, which create a loss of balance (especially in the third trimester) are a precaution that the instructor and pregnant woman should be aware of.

The format for a prenatal exercise program will vary from the traditional aerobics program in several ways. The warm-up and cooldown should be extended by two to three minutes each. The entire class should be low impact or no impact at all. A water-walking or deep-water exercise class is recommended. The stretches during the stretching segment do not need to be held quite as long as usual and should never be ballistic (bouncing). The program should not be offered in hot, humid weather. Focus should be maintained on a pelvic tilt and good body alignment.

Individuals with Arthritis

In the past, clients with arthritis have been cautioned to stay away from any movement or any type of exercise that might irritate the arthritic condition. New research has shown that the pain and stiffness in arthritic joints can be decreased through low- to moderate-intensity exercise. Movement releases synovial fluid, lubricating the joints and helping them to move more easily.

Any exercise that causes undue pain in the client with arthritis should be stopped immediately. Alternative exercises to accomplish the same goal should be used instead. Exercisers who are having an inflammatory episode, a flare-up, or who have hot joints should not participate in exercise without a physician's approval. The affected areas should be submerged beneath the water, since water naturally reduces edema (swelling). The exercise program should begin very slowly and gradually progress. Intensity and duration of exercise should be decreased. The "two-hour pain rule" should be in effect for arthritis classes: That is, if it hurts more after two hours than it did before exercise, too much was attempted. The participant should do less next time.

Format changes for arthritis classes include an elongated warm-up period to allow the synovial fluid to enter the joints and prepare for more vigorous exercise. Range-of-motion exercises are extremely important. In order to offer full-range-of-motion activities without ballistic moves, everything should be done slowly. Transitions should be fluid, with successive movements being made easily. Bouncing should be eliminated from the program. Water-walking and deep-water exercise are ideal for arthritis classes. The stretching segment should offer longer stretches, but only after the muscles have been adequately warmed. No full extensions or flexions should be incorporated into the program. While most exercise programs concentrate on using the large muscles and major joints in the body (elbows, knees, hips, etc.), this program should concentrate on the fine-motor skills and smaller joints (wrists, fingers, ankles, etc.).

The ideal water temperature for arthritic classes is 86 to 92 degrees Fahrenheit. Many arthritis participants are able to exercise in 82-degree water but find that they are more comfortable in a full unitard, wetsuit, or windsurf suit.

Individuals with Low-Back Pain

Studies show that over 80% of the American population will at some point in their lives suffer from low-back pain. Many participants come to aquatic exercise classes to take advantage of the impact-free workout afforded them. Programs need to be modified for those with low-back pain in order to ensure safety. Aquatic exercise instructors can only make modifications to alleviate the pain and protect the low back, however, since the cause of back pain can be so varied (poor posture, poor body mechanics, being overweight, poor abdominal strength, being sedentary, tight hamstrings and low back, weak gluteal muscles, tight hip flexors).

Any exercise that causes pain for low-back participants should be stopped immediately and replaced with a modified form of the movement or another that will achieve the same results without pain. The "two-hour pain rule" applies to low-back pain participants: If they hurt more two hours after class than they did before exercise, they probably attempted to do too much during the exer-cise session. They should do less next time.

Considerations in the format of the program for participants with back problems include specific strengthening and flexibility exercises. Abdominal-strengthening exercises, including isometric contractions while doing other moves, should be extensively used. Verbal cues regarding abdominals, such as "Hold the abdominals in, stand tall, remember the pelvic tilt, keep a slight flex in your knee, lift your ribs," and so on, will help the participant. Strengthening gluteals can also assist. Special stretching exercises for the low back, hamstrings, and hip flexors should be incorporated. Bouncing should be eliminated completely from the program; water-walking or deep-water exercises are ideal. Arms should be used in the water, not overhead, since doing so while moving through the water can cause instability and lumbar hyperextension. The warm-up period can be slightly elongated. Moves that involve lateral flexion, forward flexion, and spinal rotation are tolerable if used singly. Spinal flexion and rotation should not be combined, nor should lateral flexion and rotation.

Children

Exercise for children has come into the spotlight, as parents discover their children are in poor physical condition.

In comparison to adults' programs, children's programs should be modified in two ways. Namely, children differ from adults in their thermoregulatory capacity and their anaerobic capacity. Children are slightly deficient in their ability to perspire, so instructors must take special care to discourage high-intensity workouts when the pool water, air humidity, or air temperature is high. Children also are deficient in their anaerobic capacity; again, high-intensity anaerobic exercise should be discouraged.

Children's aquatic fitness programs should

follow the same format as traditional aqua-aerobics classes. Programming includes education by involving the senses (rhythm, balance), emotions (movement designed to deal with feelings and body response), creativity (conceiving images, thoughts, actions), imagery (storytelling in workout movement patterns), and relaxation training.

Children's aquatic programs should always involve interesting challenges to keep them enjoyable. Program activities should vary frequently.

All types of equipment can be used in children's aquatic classes, adding variety and challenge. Balloons, small balls, soccer balls, and beach balls can all be used, as can traditional aquatic equipment such as aqua gloves, AquaFins, HydroFit, and AquaFlex fitness paddles. All will bring variety and enjoyment to the program. Exercise bands and tubing, Frisbees, and sports equipment have also been used with success. When adding equipment to a children's program, gradual overload should be stressed to prevent injury.

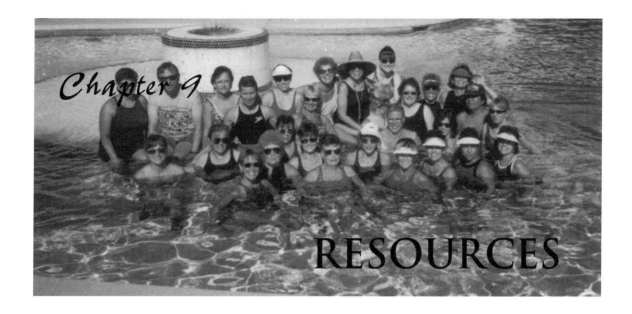

Catalogs and Equipment

Adolph Kiefer & Associates
1700 Kiefer Drive
Zion, IL 60099
Phone: 800-323-4071
Fax: 800-654-7946 / 847-746-8888
Web Site: www.kiefer.com

Aqua Gear, Inc.
13297 Temple Blvd.
West Palm Beach, FL 33412-2382
Phone: 888-426-4327 / 561-753-4636
Fax: 561-753-4697
Web Site: http://www.aqua-gear.com

Aquatic Exercise Association
P.O. Box 1609
Nokomis, FL 34274-1609
Phone: 888-AEA-WAVE (232-9283)
Fax: 941-486-8820
Web Site: www.aeawave.com

Blue Moon® Aqua Products
TRMN Enterprises, Inc.
625 Luse Drive
Columbus, OH 47201
Phone: 800-944-1176
Fax: 812-342-0743
Web Site: www.bluemoonswim.com

Fitness First Products
P.O. Box 251
Shawnee Mission, KS 66201
Phone: 800-421-1791
Fax: 800-421-0036
Web Site: www.fitness1st.com

Fitness Mart®
Country Technology, Inc.
P.O. Box 87
Gays Mills, WI 54631
Phone: 608-735-4718
Fax: 608-735-4859
Web Site: www.fitnessmart.com

Fitness Wholesale

3064 W. Edgerton
Silver Lake, OH 44224
Phone: 800-537-5512 / 330-929-7227
Web Site: www.fwonline.com

Hydro-Fit® Incorporated

1328 West 2nd Avenue
Eugene, OR 97402-4127
Phone: 541-484-4361 / 800-346-7295
Fax: 541-484-1443
Web Site: www.hydrofit.com

Hydro-Tone Fitness Systems, Inc.

16691 Gothard Street, Suite M
Huntington Beach, CA 92647
Phone: 800-622-8663 / 714-848-8284
Fax: 714-848-9035
Web Site: www.hydrotone.com

JoShel Engineering

P.O. Box 186
Oswego, NY 13126
Phone: 315-343-2857
Fax: 315-343-1318

OPTP

3700 Annapolis Lane, Suite 175
Minneapolis, MN 55447
Phone: 800-367-7393 / 612-553-0452
Fax: 612-553-9355
Web Site: www.optp.com

Pro-Fit

12012 156th Avenue SE
Renton, WA 980598-6317
Phone: 425-255-3817

Recreonics Inc.

7696 Zionsville Road
Indianapolis, IN 46268
Phone: 800-428-3254 / 502-456-5706
Fax: 502-458-9777
Web Site: www.recreonics.com

Sprint/Rothhammer

P.O. Box 3840
San Luis Obispo, CA 93403-3840
Phone: 800-235-2156
Fax: 800-652-6364 / 805-541-5339
Web Site: www.sprintaquatics.com

Water Gear

P.O. Box 759
Pismo Beach, CA 93446
Phone: 800-794-6432 / 805-343-1778
Fax: 805-343-6078
Web Site: www.watergear.com

World Wide Aquatics

10500 University Center Drive, Suite 295
Tampa, FL 33612-6462
Phone: 800-543-4459 / 813-972-0818
Fax: 813-972-0905
E-mail: info@wwaquatics.com
Web Site: www.worldwideaquatics.com

Education/Organizations

Aquatic Exercise Association

P.O. Box 1609
Nokomis, FL 34274-1609
Phone: 888-AEA-WAVE (232-9283)
Fax: 941-486-8820
Web Site: www.aeawave.com

Resources

American Alliance for Health, Physical Education, Recreation and Dance: Aquatic Council (AAHPERD)

1900 Association Drive
Reston, VA 22091
Phone: 800-213-7193 / 703-476-3400
Fax: 703-476-9527
Web Site: www.aahperd.org

Aquatic Therapy & Rehab Institute

Rt. 1, Box 218
Chassell, MI 49916-9710
Phone: 906-482-9500
Fax: 906-482-4388
Web Site: www.atri.org

National Recreation and Park Association: Aquatic Sector (NRPA)

National Aquatic Section
22377 Belmont Ridge Rd.
Ashburn, VA 20148
Phone: 703-858-0784
Fax: 703-858-0794
Web Site: www.nrpa.org

Glossary

Abduction – Movement away from the midline of the body, out of anatomical position; to move similar parts apart; the reverse movement from adduction (see Adduction).

ACSM – American College of Sports Medicine.

Adaptation – An improvement in fitness that results when the body adjusts to overload conditions; also called training.

Adduction – Movement toward the midline of the body, into anatomical position; to move similar parts together; the return movement from abduction (see Abduction).

Aerobic – Technically, that which is living or active in the presence of oxygen; generally used to describe a type of exercise that produces cardiorespiratory benefits; also the most active portion of a typical workout.

Agility – The ability to change movement rapidly, accurately, and gracefully.

Agonist – A muscle that contracts with the simultaneous lengthening action of the antagonist with which it is paired.

Antagonist – A muscle that is lengthened with the simultaneous contraction of the agonist muscle with which it is paired.

Anterior – Positioned before or toward the front of the body.

Aquatic aerobics – A type of aerobic program done in the water.

Arthritis – An inflammation of the joints.

Atrophy – The wasting away of muscle strength and size from lack of use; progressive decline.

Balance – The stability produced by an equal distribution of weight on either side of an axis; maintaining equilibrium while stationary or moving.

Ballistic – A fast, jerky, bouncing type of movement (such as stretching) that can easily cause injury.

Body composition – Overall body makeup in terms of relative proportions of lean body mass and fat.

Buoyancy – The ability to float or rise in water.

Calorie – A unit of energy, namely, that needed to raise the temperature of 1 gram of water by 1 degree Celsius. (A kilocalorie is the amount of energy needed to raise the temperature of 1 kilogram of water 1 degree Celsius.)

Cardiac cycle – The time period from one heartbeat to the next.

Cardiorespiratory endurance – The ability of the heart to supply oxygen from the respiratory system to the rest of the body during sustained exercise; one of five components of physical fitness.

Cardiorespiratory system – The body system comprised of the heart, lungs, and blood vessels (which includes the veins, arteries, and capillaries); its purpose is to carry oxygenated blood to the muscles and return deoxygenated blood to the heart; also called the cardiovascular system.

Carotid artery – One of two arteries found on the neck to either side of the throat.

Carotid pulse – The pulse felt at the carotid artery in the neck.

Circuit training – An aerobic workout combining strength training and aerobic conditioning in a variety of activities, usually completed as a series in a certain order and/or on a course.

Circumduction – Movement in a circular pattern.

Concentric contraction – The phase of contraction in which the muscle shortens; also called the positive phase (see also Eccentric contraction).

Connective tissue – Tissue such as ligaments and tendons that binds joints.

Contraindication – A condition or disease that precludes the use of a particular exercise.

Coordination – The integration of separate motor activities in the smooth, efficient execution of an activity.

Deep-water exercise – Any type of water exercise program done in water depth greater than the height of the participant.

Dive reflex – A primitive reflex that prompts lowering of the heartrate and blood pressure when the face is submerged in water; associated with a nerve found in the nasal area.

Dorsal – Positioned behind or toward the back of the body; also the top of the foot.

Dorsiflex – Flexion of the toes up toward the shin.

Drag forces – Resistant forces that cause an object to move slowly through the water.

Duration – The length of an individual workout; ACSM guidelines suggest a continuous aerobic portion of 20 to 60 minutes.

Dyspnea – Difficult or labored breathing.

Eccentric contraction – The phase of contraction in which the muscle lengthens; also called the negative phase (see also Concentric contraction).

Eddy drag – Resistance that occurs alongside an object moving through the water.

Extension – The straightening or unbending of a joint, increasing the angle between bones; the return movement from flexion (see Flexion).

Extensor – A muscle that extends a joint, generally working with gravity; usually, the weaker of the muscle pair.

Flexibility – The ability of the muscles to flex and extend the joints, providing movement through a normal range of motion; one of five components of physical fitness.

Flexion – The bending or flexing of a joint, decreasing the angle between bones; the opposite of extension (see Extension).

Flexor – A muscle that bends or flexes a joint, generally working against gravity; usually, the stronger of the muscle pair.

Footstrike – The foot hitting a surface.

Frequency – The number of times a workout is repeated, usually in terms of hours per week.

Frontal resistance – Resistance that occurs in front an object moving through the water.

Hydrostatic pressure – The pressure exerted by any fluid on any body at rest.

Hyperextension – Moving a joint past anatomical position.

Immersion – Putting a limb or the body into the water.

Inertia – The physical principle that a mass tends to resist changes in speed or direction of motion.

Intensity – The degree of challenge a workout poses for the cardiorespiratory system.

Interval training – An exertive exercise program, combining high-intensity segments with moderate- or low-intensity segments.

Joint – A place where two bones are joined, usually (although not exclusively) to allow motion; also called an articulation.

Joint capsule – The ligaments, tendons, membranes, articular surfaces, and cartilage that surround a joint.

Karvonen formula – A mathematical formula used to determine target heartrate.

Laminar – The quality of being streamlined or flat.

Lateral – Positioned away from the midline of the body, toward the outside.

Lateral flexion (of the spine) – Bending the torso toward the outside; generally used to describe sidebends.

Law of leverage – The physical principle that states that the length of the lever determines the force needed to move it; short levers require less force than long ones.

Ligament – The strong, fibrous tissue that connects bones.

Maximal heartrate – The greatest number of times per minute the heart is capable of beating.

Maximum working heartrate – The upper end of the working heartrate range (see Working heartrate range); the maximum number of times the heart should beat per minute during exercise for cardiorespiratory training to take place.

Medial – Positioned toward the midline of the object or body.

Metabolic rate – The level at which physical and chemical demands are processed in the body, providing energy for life support; regular exercise enhances metabolic rate.

Minimum working heartrate – The lower end of the working heartrate range (see Working heartrate range); the minimum number of times the heart should beat per minute during exercise for cardiorespiratory training to take place.

Mode – The type of exercise selected for a cardiorespiratory workout; the optimal mode is based on large-muscle activity, maintained continuously and rhythmical in nature.

Muscle balance – The condition achieved when the muscles in a muscle pair have equal strength and flexibility.

Muscular endurance – The ability of a muscle to repeat a contraction with a moderate workload over a sustained period of time; one of five components of physical fitness.

Muscular strength – The ability of a muscle to exert great force in a single effort, usually achieved by lifting weights; one of five components of physical fitness.

Musculoskeletal fatigue – Fatigue brought on by the overuse of any muscle; characterized by pain in a bone, joint, or muscle.

Obesity – The condition of having an excessive level of body fat (approximately 25% for men and 33% for women), usually in combination with being overweight; frequently results in significant health impairment.

Optimum working heartrate – The middle portion of the working heartrate range (see Working heartrate range); the ideal number of times the heart should beat per minute during exercise for cardiorespiratory training to take place; varies with fitness goal.

Osteoporosis – A condition characterized by loss of bone mineral due to calcium deficiency; a potentially crippling condition that often afflicts older women.

Overtraining – An excessive level of exercise frequency, duration, or intensity, causing fatigue and/or injury.

Overuse injury – A physical problem caused by putting too much stress on one area of the body over a long period of time.

Oxygen consumption – The rate at which oxygen is used to produce energy for cellular work; also called oxygen uptake; used to measure exercise intensity or energy expenditure (the more efficient the consumption, the greater the level of fitness).

Perceived exertion – An individualís ability to judge the intensity at which he is exercising.

Periodization – A method of joining physiological conditioning with technique learning; both short- and long-term fitness goals are established; to be achieved by various programs over cycles of different lengths (i.e., six months, several months, a week).

Physiological – Characteristic of or appropriate to a bodyís normal functioning.

Plantar – Positioned along the bottom surface, such as the sole of the foot.

Plantarflex – Flexion in which the toes are pointed toward the floor (as in ballet).

Plyometric – A type of exercise characterized by a series of jumping, bounding, and hopping moves; doing so preloads and forces the stretching of the muscle immediately prior to concentric action.

Posterior – Positioned toward the back (dorsal) side of the body.

Poststretch – The flexibility segment of the workout that occurs after the aerobic portion; helps the muscles relax and return to their normal resting state.

Power – In fitness terms, transferring energy into force at a fast rate; a combination of strength and speed in one explosive action.

Prestretch – The flexibility segment of the workout that occurs after the thermal warm-up but before activities requiring high intensity and full range of motion.

Progressive overload – A philosophy of exercise that purports that the body (or one of its systems) will adapt to meet an increase in the demand made on it, resulting in improved physical fitness; in terms of physical conditioning, the level of demand should be controlled and increase gradually; also called progressive resistance.

Pronation – Turning the palms down or the soles of the feet out to the sides.

Prone – Positioned lying face down.

Proprioception – The reception of stimuli generated from within oneís body.

Reaction time – The amount of time that elapses between stimulation and response to that stimulation.

Recovery heartrate – The number of times the heart beats per minute when monitored 5 to 10 minutes after vigorous exercise; an indication of how quickly the cardiorespiratory system is able to return to its pre-exercise condition, which is a reflection of fitness.

Repetitions – The number of times a particular movement is repeated during a set (see Set); also called reps.

Resistance – The load, force, or weight applied against the muscle.

Respiration rate – The number of breaths taken per minute.

Resting heartrate – The number of times the heart beats per minute when the body is at rest; the average is 72; a low resting heartrate usually indicates fitness.

Reversibility – The principle that fitness benefits cannot be stored by the body but must be maintained through regular exercise; training levels begin to decline after several days of inactivity.

Rotation – Turning on an axis; spinal rotation is twisting to the right and then to the left.

Rotator – A type of muscle that serves to rotate a part of the body.

Set – A number of movement repetitions performed in sequence (see Repetitions); a rest period is allowed between sets to allow the muscles to recover.

Shallow-water jogging – Jogging in waist- to chest-deep water at a fast enough pace to cause the necessary overload for cardiorespiratory benefits.

Skeletal system – The bodyís framework of bones and how they function in supporting tissues and protecting organs.

Skeleton – The assembly of bones.

Specificity – The principle that states that only that part of the body being exercised according to progressive overload will adapt and improve (see also Progressive overload).

Speed – The act or state of moving quickly.

Sport-specific workout – A type of aerobic program designed to train athletes in a specific sport, such as bicycling or tennis; emphasis is on developing the muscle strength, flexibility, and skills specific to the given sport.

Static stretch – A type of stretch in which the extended position is held without bouncing to increase muscle flexibility.

Streamlined – Characterized by contoured physical qualities such that movement through water causes very little resistance; resistance is proportional to velocity.

Stretch reflex – A type of reflex that causes the muscle fibers to contract when a stretch is begun; may result in muscle tears if ballistic stretching is used, which is why static stretching is recommended (see Ballistic; Static stretching).

Stroke volume – The amount of blood the heart pumps in one contraction.

Submaximal – Employing about 60% of the maximum ability of the heart or a muscle group; working out at this level increases cardiovascular endurance and/or muscular strength.

Supination – Turning the palms upward or rolling the soles of the feet in, toward each other.

Synovial fluid – The transparent, viscous, and lubricating fluid secreted by the membranes of articulations, bursa, and tendon sheaths; enhances movement.

Synovial membrane – The thin, silklike film encasing a joint.

Talk test – A method of testing workout intensity; namely, an individual should work out at an intensity that enables her to talk while exercising.

Target zone – The range on a scale of heartrate – delineated by the minimum and maximum working heartrates – that represents the appropriate intensity for safe and effective exercise; also called the working heartrate range, target heartrate range, or training zone (see Maximum working heartrate; Minimum working heartrate).

Tendon – A fibrous band that connects muscle to bone.

Thermal warm-up – The initial segment of the workout in which the muscles are gradually stimulated; this increases the muscles' demand for oxygen and releases synovial fluid into the joints.

Thermoregulatory system – The body system that regulates the core temperature.

Toning – The segment of the workout that develops muscular endurance.

Torque – A type of force or combination of forces that produces twisting or rotation.

Transverse abduction/adduction – Abduction and adduction done across the body; also called horizontal abduction/adduction. (Transverse abduction is when the leg is straight, the hip is flexed, and one leg moves laterally toward the outside of the body; transverse adduction is when the leg is straight, the hip is flexed, and one leg moves laterally to the inside, across the other.)

Turbidity – The state of being murky or cloudy (e.g., after sentiments have been stirred up).

Turbulent – The disruptive movement through water produced when an object encounters extreme resistance because it is not streamlined; resistance is proportional to velocity squared.

VO_2 max – The level of maximal oxygen consumption.

Variability – The principle that adaptation or fitness improvements are enhanced by varying the intensity, length, or type of workout.

Ventral – The front surface of the body.

Vital capacity – The measurement of lung capacity; depressed by hydrostatic pressure.

Water walking – Striding in waist- to chest-deep water at a pace fast enough to create the necessary overload for cardiorespiratory benefits.

Working heartrate range – The range on a scale of heartrate – delineated by the minimum and maximum working heartrates – that represents the appropriate intensity for safe and effective exercise; also called the target zone, target heartrate range, or training zone (see Maximum working heartrate; Minimum working heartrate).

Zero-to-peak – A mathematical formula for determining heartrate range; also called the maximal heartrate formula.

DSL, Ltd.

1218 Noridge Trail, Port Washington, WI 53074 USA
PHONE 262-284-2542   FAX 262-284-7039

Other Ruth Sova Products:

AQUATICS: The Complete Reference Guide for Aquatic Fitness Professionals	$ 54.95	_____
Aquatics Handbook	$ 22.95	_____
Aquatic Exercise	$ 19.95	_____
AQUATICS Study Guide	$ 18.95	_____
Painless Strategic Planning	$ 19.95	_____
Water Fitness After 40	$ 15.95	_____
BackHab - The Water Way to Mobility and Pain Free Living	$ 18.95	_____
BackHab Video	$ 19.95	_____
Ai Chi - Flowing Aquatic Energy	$ 12.95	_____
Ai Chi -Flowing Aquatic Energy Video	$ 19.95	_____
Ai Chi – Balance, Harmony and Healing	$ 23.95	_____
Ai Chi Mystical Music Cassette	$ 14.95	_____
Ai Chi Synchrony Cassette	$ 14.95	_____
Ai Chi Visualization Journey Cassette	$ 14.95	_____
Ai Chi Physical Focus Cassette	$ 14.95	_____
Ai Chi Laminate	$ 4.95	_____
Ai Chi Ne Laminate	$ 4.95	_____
Aqua Challenge Package	$ 29.95	_____
Life: The Burning Issues Video	$ 19.95	_____
Prunes, Carrots, and Ripples Video	$ 19.95	_____
Prunes, Carrots, and Ripples Audio Cassette	$ 9.95	_____
Positive Affirmation Daily Calendar	$ 8.95	_____
Shipping and handling		$ 4.00
Total		$ _____

Foreign customers only, please check your shipping preference: Surface mail_____   Air mail_____
Any additional shipping charges will be billed to you.

Name_____

Shipping Address_____

_____

Daytime Phone _____

U.S. Funds Only:
Check enclosed_____ Amount_____
or MC/VISA (circle one) #
_____Exp._____
Signature _____

About the Author

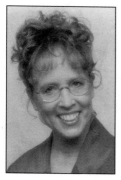

*R*uth *Sova, M.S,* an internationally known speaker, author and consultant, is founder of six successful businesses including the Aquatic Therapy and Rehab Institute, the Aquatic Exercise Association, Living Right Magazine, America's Certification Trainers, Armchair Aerobics Inc., and the Fitness Firm. A leader in the health and wellness industry, Ruth also draws on her vast experience as an entrepreneur to teach others what it takes to assume the risk of business and enterprise. Ruth serves on the Wisconsin Governor's Council on Physical Fitness and has written many articles as well as eleven books on her specialties of wellness and business.

Ruth has received:

Governor's Entrepreneurial Award
Suomi College Entrepreneurial Award
IDEA Outstanding Business Person Award
AEA Contribution to the Industry Award
CNCA Merit Award
AAHPERD Honor and Service Awards
AHA Outstanding Fund Raising Award
Wisconsin State Assembly Commendation
Key to the City of Port Washington, Wisconsin
Commemorative First Presidential Sports Award - Aquatic Exercise
Sevier-McCahill Disability International Foundation Award
Sara's City Workout Aquatic Instructor of the Year
John Williams, Jr. International Swimming Hall of Fame Adapted Aquatics Award

Ruth and her husband Bud live in Port Washington where they hike, boat, and regularly kill their houseplants. Their 30+ years of marriage has produced two children, Nicole and Kurt, one son-in-law, Dave, one daughter-in-law, Erin, and one cat, Captain Tony (hardier than the plants). Ruth believes that we should all eat real cheese, real ice cream, and real butter to keep the Wisconsin dairy industry strong.